UN9
WHO
88E17

MO-DOF

C0-BPA-572

Economic Support
for National
Health for All
Strategies

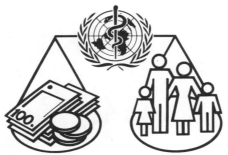

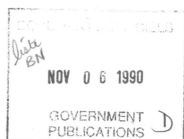

liste
BN

NOV 0 6 1990

GOVERNMENT
PUBLICATIONS

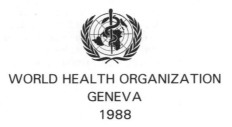

WORLD HEALTH ORGANIZATION
GENEVA
1988

ISBN 92 4 156122 X

© World Health Organization 1988

Publications of the World Health Organization enjoy copyright protection in accordance with the provisions of Protocol 2 of the Universal Copyright Convention. For rights of reproduction or translation of WHO publications, in part or *in toto*, application should be made to the Office of Publications, World Health Organization, Geneva, Switzerland. The World Health Organization welcomes such applications.

The designations employed and the presentation of the material in this publication do not imply the expression of any opinion whatsoever on the part of the Secretariat of the World Health Organization concerning the legal status of any country, territory, city or area or of its authorities, or concerning the delimitation of its frontiers or boundaries.

The mention of specific companies or of certain manufacturers' products does not imply that they are endorsed or recommended by the World Health Organization in preference to others of a similar nature that are not mentioned. Errors and omissions excepted, the names of proprietary products are distinguished by initial capital letters.

PRINTED IN SWITZERLAND

88/7590-PCL-5000

Contents

Foreword

This publication is the outcome of a series of activities, including studies, consultations and meetings, designed to clarify issues and identify options for optimum mobilization and use of resources in actions aimed at achieving health for all. These activities provided a substantial input to the Technical Discussions held during the Fortieth World Health Assembly (May 1987) on economic support for national health for all strategies. During these Discussions a number of important recommendations were made (see Chapter VI) which formed the basis for resolution WHA40.30, adopted by the Fortieth World Health Assembly.

Resolution WHA40.30 adopted by the Fortieth World Health Assembly, May 1987

Economic support for national health-for-all strategies

The Fortieth World Health Assembly,

Appreciating the outcome of the Technical Discussions held at the Fortieth World Health Assembly on economic support for national health-for-all strategies, and recalling resolution WHA39.22 on the Technical Discussions held during the Thirty-ninth World Health Assembly;

Reaffirming that health is an integral part of development and is therefore the responsibility of the health sector, other related sectors, the individual and the community in general;

Further reaffirming that the goal of health for all can only be achieved through primary health care, which requires major reorientation of policies and perspectives in the way health is perceived, protected, provided and delivered;

Aware that the prevailing adverse trends in the world economy, aggravated in the developing countries by the formidable burden of servicing external debts and the deterioration of the balance of trade, jeopardize the possibilities of many countries to reach the goal of health for all by the year 2000;

Stressing the need for continued political leadership and determination in the face of these adverse trends in order to achieve the goal of health for all in the spirit of social equity;

Mindful of the need to intensify action to increase economic support for national strategies for health for all and in particular to mobilize and utilize health resources, with emphasis on social relevance, equity, managerial efficiency and effectiveness;

1. URGES Member States:

   (1) to continue to ensure that the health of the most disadvantaged and vulnerable population groups is protected when economic adjustment policies are designed and implemented;

   (2) to consider the responsibilities and contributions of all potential partners in health development, including health-related sectors, the community, social security agencies, nongovernmental organizations, and the private sector, when developing national health-for-all strategies, and to establish appropriate mechanisms to achieve their maximum involvement and collaboration in financing health development;

(3)   to review their current patterns of resource allocation in the health sector and reorient as appropriate their spending priorities, including allocation of any additional resources for the provision of primary health care, giving preferential attention to the underserved and the neediest segments of population;

(4)   to strengthen the capacity of local bodies to mobilize, channel and allocate resources and ensure that monies raised by health services remain at the disposal of the health sector;

(5)   to take urgent steps to reduce waste and increase efficient use of resources through technical and administrative decentralization, better management, information and supervision;

(6)   to pay particular attention to the choice of technologies appropriate to each level of the health care system with a view to improving efficiency and effectiveness, and develop methods for cost control with due regard to maintaining the quality of care;

(7)   to encourage more rational use of drugs, thereby avoiding misuse and wastage of resources;

(8)   to establish a programme for better management and maintenance of equipment through appropriate procedures, training of personnel, and ensuring the availability of spare parts;

(9)   to pay special attention to health manpower development in order to raise appreciation of the need for efficiency and cost control through new and innovative teaching/learning experiences which concentrate on *in situ* problem-solving methods and the use of practical health system research;

(10)   to establish realistically the costs of implementing their national health-for-all strategies and plans which reflect national priorities, paying particular attention to future recurrent costs, to identify the means of closing any gaps between resources required and available, and to review health policies and strategies with the joint involvement of ministries of health, planning, finance and other relevant ministries;

(11)   to evaluate the adequacy of existing revenue-raising measures and to explore new financing options consistent with the overall goals of equity and effectiveness;

(12)   to strengthen their capacities in financial planning and management at all levels, particularly at the district level, through training in financial analysis, health economics and financial planning and management; by strengthening management information systems; and by incorporating research and economic analysis as an important input in the process of decision-making;

(13)   to consider regulatory measures that will be effective in controlling cost increase and maintaining an acceptable level of quality in the health services, public and private;

(14) to promote individual responsibility for health through the adoption of healthy life-styles and other measures which protect their population from avoidable health risks, thereby also reducing the future financial burden on the health care system;

(15) to publicize their health plans to get public understanding and support;

(16) to focus on the education of the public in the appropriate use of health care services, paying special attention to the role of women in health and health care, and optimizing the use of the mass media in such educational activities;

2. APPEALS again to the developed countries to increase their cooperation with, and assistance to, developing countries through bilateral and multilateral channels, including WHO, in implementing their national health-for-all strategies, in a spirit of self-reliance, mutual respect and social equity in the international economic field;

3. CALLS upon international and bilateral agencies to increase their support to developing countries to accelerate the implementation of national strategies for health for all, and in particular to help strengthen national capacities in research and development, in economic analysis and in financial planning and management;

4. REQUESTS the Director-General:

(1) to publish the report of the Technical Discussions on this issue and disseminate it widely to governments, organizations and agencies of the United Nations system, academic institutions and other intergovernmental, nongovernmental and voluntary organizations;

(2) to continue to monitor the impact of economic trends and policies on the health status of the most disadvantaged and vulnerable groups, and to help Member States to identify ways of mitigating their adverse repercussions;

(3) to promote the exchange of information and experiences among countries on approaches and options being used for expanding domestic economic support for health for all and for the optimum use of their resources;

(4) to give further guidance to countries on methodologies and potentialities of using different options for financing;

(5) to intensify technical cooperation with Member States to improve national capabilities in financial planning and management and economic analysis of health strategies, through relevant training and research activities, including the strengthening of centres for such training and research in developing countries;

(6) to review and strengthen as appropriate WHO capacity at regional and global levels to provide the required technical support to countries in financial

planning and management and in economic analysis of their health policies and strategies, and to mobilize additional resources for intensifying such support;

(7)   to include in progress reports on the implementation of the health-for-all strategy, in-depth reviews of efforts within countries to obtain economic support for their national strategies, including the use of nationally relevant indicators related to resource allocation.

Executive summary

Ten years ago, the World Health Assembly decided that the main social target of governments and of WHO should be the attainment by all the people of the world by the year 2000 of a level of health that would permit them to lead socially and economically productive lives. People must be healthy to contribute to and share in social and economic development and, conversely, development goals cannot be achieved without a healthy population. The historic International Conference on Primary Health Care in Alma-Ata, USSR (1978) charted a new course for the health of the citizens of the world. The Conference called for a new approach to health and health care to shrink the gap between the "haves" and "have-nots" and to achieve a more equitable distribution of health resources. The Conference further affirmed that the primary health care approach was essential to an acceptable level of health throughout the world and acknowledged that this could be attained through fuller and better use of the world's resources.

Primary health care is essential health care made accessible at a cost the country and community can afford, with methods that are practical, scientifically sound, and socially acceptable. Everyone in the community should have access to it and everyone should be involved in it. Governments together with the World Health Organization in a spirit of social justice have endorsed primary health care as the key to attaining the goal of health for all by the year 2000.

The Global Strategy for Health for All, adopted by the Thirty-fourth World Health Assembly (1981), stressed the close and complex links that exist between health and socioeconomic development. Health not only results from genuine socioeconomic development, as distinct from mere economic growth, it is also an essential investment in such development. The achievement of health goals is determined to a large extent by policies that lie outside the health sector and in particular the socioeconomic development policies. The Strategy therefore emphasized the mutual reinforcement of related policies. These principles were reaffirmed during the Technical Discussions on intersectoral action for health (1986), which further clarified the essential elements of equity-oriented development strategies and the respective roles of the crucial development sectors such as agriculture, education and environment in promoting and contributing to health goals. The Technical Discussions also highlighted the health-related policy components in the crucial development sectors.

Political determination for health for all

The overall efforts of governments to develop their health systems in response to their national health strategies has been encouraging, as was revealed by the first report on the evaluation of the Global Strategy for Health for All (1986). A high level of political will is evident. There is a growing awareness of the need for change in health systems. In some countries impressive efforts have been made to expand the health services infrastructure. Some innovative approaches to reach underserved population groups and to strengthen community-based health services are also noted. The overall benefits, however, have sometimes been less than expected because of factors such as political instability, natural disasters, and high population growth. In addition, the intervening decade has been marked by economic instability that has greatly impeded social progress in many parts of the world.

Implications of the economic climate for health for all

The global economic situation has changed drastically for the worse since 1977 when the goal of health for all was adopted. The past eight years have been the most turbulent times for the world economy in over half a century. The recession has had important implications for adjustment policies which governments have had to adopt in order to maintain a reasonable balance between economic growth and social development. This has not been an easy task for a majority of the developing countries, especially the poorest countries of the world. The health budgets of many countries have been severely reduced at a time when additional resources are required to build and sustain national health systems based on primary health care to meet the priority health needs of all people, especially the vulnerable and the underserved.

The acceptance of the goal of health for all was accompanied by the fundamental concept of equity in

health. Making quality health care available at an affordable level, however, remains a distant prospect in many countries. Aspects such as the impact of available health care, as well as concerns with efficiency and cost-benefits, are being balanced by countries against a more equitable distribution of health-related resources in order to bring health care to the vulnerable groups of their societies. The danger inherent in this balancing act is that concern with equity can give way to concern for "cost-containment" which, in practice, can be translated to mean reductions in the social expenditures for those who need them most. The manner in which the health goal is incorporated into the overall strategy as a goal of development also affects the allocation of resources and, in turn, the issue of equity.

But external economic factors cannot be entirely blamed for the under-achievement in the health sector. Many governments have not seriously taken up the strategic actions required to generate and mobilize all possible resources for health. Very few countries have attempted to make an estimate of the magnitude of resources required for their national strategies to achieve the goal of health for all. Altogether, very few *new* initiatives have been undertaken to mobilize resources internally which can have national impact. Few countries have been able to reallocate their existing health budgets preferentially to primary health care. Inefficient use of existing health resources persists; effective actions to reduce waste or to improve cost-effectiveness have been too few to have a substantial positive impact on the resource situation. The health sector remains a "weak partner" in influencing socioeconomic development policies or in mobilizing effective support from other related sectors for health activities.

Economic support for health for all

How to finance health plans and how to make the best use of resources have both become critical issues in progress towards the attainment of health for all. While financial cutbacks present major problems in the short term, in the long term the search for additional and new resources, *particularly domestic resources,* and making the most efficient use of all available resources offer the best options for financing health for all. Improved financial planning and management and bold administrative and organizational measures will also be required. The strengthening of national capability, especially that of the ministries of health or equivalent bodies, in developing and implementing policies based on sound economic analysis and strong financial management, will be a prerequisite to effective national action.

The purpose of this book is to focus attention on the options for strengthening and expanding economic support for national strategies for health for all. It suggests that five broad needs ought to be addressed. These needs are: (i) to project the financial requirements imposed by national health policies and to assess the capacity of currently available revenue measures to meet those needs; (ii) to evaluate the quality of resource mobilization efforts in terms of their equity, adequacy, reliability, impact on the supply and demand for services, and ease of administration; (iii) to increase the productivity of the resources available to governments by focusing attention on efficiency and cost-effectiveness of activities undertaken by the health sector; (iv) to reappraise the roles and responsibilities of potential partners in health, including the government, community, nongovernmental organizations and the private sector; and (v) to strengthen national capability in formulating and implementing sound economic policies and approaches in support of national strategies for health for all.

Planning and managing the finances

The elaboration of a well-defined plan of action, including a financial master plan, is an essential part of the strategy for attaining health for all. The financial implications of declared health policies need to be assessed carefully. Financial master planning can provide a framework for assessing the feasibility of implementing the plan of action against the resource availability. It can identify the resource gap and suggest options to close this gap, including either increasing resource availability or modifying the implementation objectives.

Such plans would estimate the capital and recurrent costs of implementing the countrywide programmes included in the proposed plan of action and would identify sources of funds to meet these requirements. The process seeks to identify the boundaries within which a health plan could be implemented. Among the essential steps are: estimating the costs of meeting proclaimed health goals and distributing these costs over a period of time between the initiation of the plan and the year 2000; comparing recurrent costs with the revenues likely to become available from existing sources of finance; exploring all possible sources of finance; and reconciling planned expenditure with the revenue both from existing and further sources of finance. If resource gaps exist, either the plan of action should be modified or mechanisms to mobilize new resources should be suggested.

While a financial master plan will help to establish the extent to which a policy can be implemented, programme budgeting is required to enhance the efficiency and effectiveness of implementation. The budgeting system should stress the links between programme objectives and the use of resources and the relationships between capital expenditures and recurrent costs.

Sound financial planning and management are thus essential to the implementation of national health for all strategies. Decisions on mechanisms to finance health plans are inevitably political. The task of planners is essentially to develop options for political decision-making. Ministers of health need to encourage their planning staff to engage in creative thinking, even if some of the options presented prove to be politically unacceptable.

Mobilizing resources

The desired increases in coverage, and the maintenance and improvement of content and quality of health services, will require additional resources in many countries. Available government revenues in most cases will not be sufficient to cover the requirements. New and alternative options will have to be considered. Strategies for financing health for all will no doubt reflect the various characteristics of national economies.

In choosing a strategy, however, certain criteria should be applied. These include equity, adequacy, reliability, impact on supply and demand, intersectoral nature, and administrative feasibility.

Many options for financing health services are now being widely considered. First, governments may pay for health care from public revenues. This requires that additional resources be allocated for health activities. Second, employers and employees may be required to contribute to a health insurance scheme, or employers can provide health services for their employees. Third, institutions, publicly or privately owned, may be created to attract voluntary insurance contributions and to dispense these revenues to providers of health services. Fourth, schemes of community financing may be developed. Fifth, consumers may be required to pay for part of the cost of the health services they use. Many variations of these options are being devised. Each of these options has distinctive economic, financial, political, and administrative attributes which need to be carefully examined.

Making better use of resources

There is general concern in all countries that the available resources are not being used most effectively or efficiently. A large share of health resources is wasted because of poor managerial practices and use of inappropriate technologies or human resources. Making better use of resources implies improved accountability, increased efficiency in the allocation and utilization of resources, and effective means of cost-containment.

Accountability can be improved by strengthening formal accounting and management information systems and by providing adequate and supportive supervision. Resource wastage due to misappropriation, underemployment or deterioration must be given serious attention by health managers. In many cases communities can also be more actively involved in the management of resources at the local level. They will need to be supported in this task by the central levels.

Efficiency in the use of resources can be enhanced by several means. If access to health services were more equitable, cost-efficiency would generally be greater. The cost to the providers as well as to the individuals must be considered. Many options are available for achieving greater efficiency in the use of human resources. The main objective should be to make rational use of health personnel consistent with the functions of each level of the health system. Appropriate training and supervision would need to be provided to ensure quality and performance. Individuals and families can be informed and educated to take a greater share of responsibility for their health. Careful choice of technologies appropriate to each level of the health care system would also serve to increase efficiency. Cost-effective strategies can be applied to specific health problems and, finally, the strengthening of management support services would be crucial to sustain efficient delivery of health services.

Cost-containment policies have begun to emerge, particularly in many developed countries. Many new approaches are being applied to influence both the supply and the demand of health services. These have included a revision of reimbursable fee scales, an imposition of user charges and a regulation of the content of care through review committees. Public education and information on these aspects is also receiving considerable attention. An informed public can be a valuable asset.

Responsibilities and institutional relationships

Health care is a shared responsibility which rests upon the individual, the community and the government. Within the government responsibility, health goals have to be incorporated as part of the sectoral goals of many different sectors including health, environment, education, agriculture, and housing. Given the magnitude of the task of attaining health for all, and particularly of securing adequate economic support for this, concerted and coordinated action at all levels is indispensable. Collective commitment of all concerned is required in order to ensure the equitable distribution of resources for health care.

A lack of information precludes a thorough analysis of the respective share of the responsibility and contribution of the different entities involved in health matters. But it is clear that, in many developed and developing countries, the public sector controls only a portion of the overall resources available for health care. While no blueprint can be applicable for organizing the institutional relationships of the different entities or subsystems involved in health matters, it is clear that greater coherence needs to be achieved among these subsystems and that all subsystems should reflect primary health care as their major goal.

Collaboration between various institutions and agencies is essential and should be based on a clear allocation of responsibilities in order to ensure the most efficient use of resources. Countries need to examine what is the feasible organizational framework in their own national situation that would enhance such collaboration.

Strengthening national capability

Mobilizing economic support for health for all has many implications for national health policy-makers and health administrators. The policy-makers in health need to be strong advocates for promoting social priorities in economic adjustment policies. They must mobilize commitment and support from other sectors, especially those closely related to health. The health administrators must increase their capability in defining equitable schemes of financing and of allocation of resources. They must be able to provide policy-makers with different options for mobilizing additional resources. And finally, they must manage their scarce resources optimally and efficiently.

These implications also suggest the need for substantive improvements in information for health planning and management, for the development of capacity for research, processing and analysing economic data, and for the acceptance by senior managers and policy-makers of the importance of these new inputs into the process of decision-making.

Technical capability in the health sector in these areas will require considerable strengthening in most developing countries.

Conclusions

The goal of health for all by the year 2000 has been called ambitious. Those who regard it as such disregard the fundamental principles embodied in the primary health care approach, which is the key to achieving the goal.

Primary health care emphasizes health as an integral part of development and, thus a responsibility of not just what is traditionally defined as the health sector, but of people, other related sectors and the community in general. Primary health care calls for the use of affordable, relevant and socially acceptable technologies, and requires that the strengthening or building up of the health infrastructure should begin in the home and at the community level, the other levels of the health system being supportive to these.

Respect for these principles requires a major reorientation of policies and perspectives in the way health is perceived, protected, and promoted.

These principles also apply to resource allocation and distribution policies. A concern for the care and protection of the poor and the disadvantaged groups, the according of high priorities to prevention and promotive actions, and the use of inexpensive yet effective technologies to provide at least the eight essential elements of primary health care, should be reflected in such policies if choices and sacrifices have to be made. Resource allocation policies have to take into account not just what goes to health care, but also what goes to other important determinants of health such as education, environment, and food, again with due considerations for principles of equity.

The issue is not where the money is going to come from to pay for health care, but rather what broad policy framework is required to expand the economic support for health for all. This support must come from individuals, families, communities, the private sector, nongovernmental sectors and, of course, government sources. The issue is not just what extra resources will be required and how to mobilize them, but also how those resources that are available can be used most efficiently and productively.

Analysis of economic support for health for all should not be clouded by a narrow vision of financing primary health care or medical care by the public or private sector. It should encompass the policy and institutional frameworks that will provide a coherent strategy for the full, active and mutually reinforcing participation of all potential partners. No one should be allowed to escape this responsibility. This is not just a political or social dream, it is an economic challenge.

Achieving health for all will require sacrifices. The mechanisms and methods used to finance and support services will continue to be imperfect. The task of finding long-term solutions is difficult but must be faced if the health of the future generations is not to be jeopardized.

Introduction

The world economic situation has changed drastically for the worse since 1977 when the goal of health for all was adopted. The health budgets of many countries have been severely reduced at a time when additional resources are required to build and sustain national health systems based on primary health care to meet the priority needs of all people, especially the underserved. The reductions in the health budgets have tended to affect key items such as drugs, equipment, communications and transport, seriously jeopardizing the delivery of essential health care in rural areas. Policies and plans that have been approved in principle at the highest government level have not been fully implemented.

The adjustment policies adopted by governments in times of economic crisis, as in the recent widespread economic recession, are important indicators of the priority that health care receives in the national allocation or resources. Often when resources are constrained, the relatively low priority for health in resource allocation and the neglect of the social costs of adjustments become pronounced.

Economic support for health for all

It was recognized at the outset that to carry out the Global Strategy for Health for All would mean generating and mobilizing all possible resources. This implied first of all making the most efficient use of existing resources both within and among countries. At the same time, additional resources would need to be generated. Among actions specified for providing economic support for health for all were: careful analysis of the resource needs for the provision of primary health care, particularly for underserved population groups; consideration of the benefit of various health programmes in relation to the cost, as well as the effectiveness of different technologies and different ways of organizing the health system in relation to the cost; estimation of the order of magnitude of the total financial needs to implement the national strategy up to the year 2000; and consideration of alternative ways of financing the health system, including mobilizing domestic and external resources.

There is evidence to suggest that governments as a whole have not yet given serious and in-depth consideration to these strategic actions. Very few countries have costed their plans for health for all, let alone identified sources from which they can be financed. Some plans that were costed before the worst effects of the economic recession were known now seem to be over-ambitious. Altogether, very few new initiatives have been undertaken to mobilize resources internally which can have national impact. Few countries have been successful in reallocating their existing health budgets preferentially to primary health care. The role of the private sector in national health for all strategies has not been fully defined. Even in countries where recent economic improvements have been noted at the individual and family levels, the role of the individuals in sharing the cost of health care has not been reconsidered. With the economic problems affecting the developed countries as well, the anticipated increases in health aid from rich countries to the poor have not materialized.

How to finance health plans and how to make the best use of resources have both become critical issues in progress towards the attainment of health for all. While financial cutbacks present major problems in the short term, it is nevertheless true that, in the long term, the search for additional resources, including new cost-sharing mechanisms, can provide countries with fresh opportunities to look again at how they are using their existing resources. The pros and cons of strategic options for ensuring the future funding of the total capital investment costs and the implied increasing burden of recurrent expenditure are worthy of analysis. Also, the health policies, the financial management measures and the administrative and organizational structures may need to be reviewed for possible adjustments.

Scope of the publication

This publication explores the critical issues in the planning and management of the financing of the health sector. It also presents and analyses alternatives for mobilizing additional economic support for national health for all strategies and addresses the measures for obtaining maximum impact from health resources, with emphasis on social relevance, equity and efficiency. Finally, it explores responsibilities and institutional relationships in economic support for health for all.

No attempt has been made in this book to cover the entire spectrum of issues. To help Member States to address, practically, the economic implications of attaining health for all in a spirit of self-reliance, and as a complement to the 1986 Technical Discussions on intersectoral action for health, a deliberate effort has been made to concentrate essentially on one vital aspect, namely *domestic resources*. This does not mean that the question of external resources will not be considered. However, the emphasis will be mainly on the implications of the use of domestic resources on the sustainability of activities initiated, when countries have to support fully their operating costs.

Given the complexity of issues and the diversity of country and sector situations, no pretension is made of giving a particular set of prescriptions for effective health financing nor is it suggested that there are universally applicable ways of solving the problem of health financing. The intention is to present a balanced picture of potential measures.

The world economic climate and its implications for health for all
Chapter I describes the global economic climate and its implications for the health sector. Within this macroeconomic context, health sector issues to cope with financial problems are pointed out in terms of equity, efficiency and quality of health care. The need for economic support for pursuing equity-oriented health policies is emphasized.

Planning and managing the finances

Chapter II focuses on improved financial management as a way of increasing the effectiveness of available resources. Financial planning is described as a device for determining the financial feasibility and sustainability of strategies and strengthening the health sector's position when requesting funds in the future. Programme budgeting is discussed as a tool for controlling the use of resources. Accounting practices are reviewed to improve fiscal management. Lastly, economic analysis to ensure adequate financing arrangements is explored.

Mobilizing resources

Chapter III presents alternative ways of mobilizing financial resources at the community and national levels for health systems based on primary health care. These include insurance schemes, community financing, cost-sharing and other mechanisms. The criteria by which alternatives might be evaluated are provided. These methods determine the ability of the sector to cope with financial uncertainty to meet particular needs such as importation of drugs and spare parts. Thus the chapter analyses the capacity of different mechanisms to generate funds in order to meet needs for foreign exchange, to accommodate growth in demand, to absorb price inflation, and to service the contractual obligations of the sector.

Making better use of resources

Chapter IV addresses the measures for obtaining the maximum impact from health resources with emphasis on social relevance, equity, efficiency, and cost-effectiveness. The chapter first discusses ways of reducing waste in the use of all health resources and mechanisms for improving accountability. It then presents a framework for the efficiency of health services at all levels. Alternatives for cost-effective access to health care and strategies, including the use of appropriate technology and manpower mixes, are examined. Measures for cost-control and cost-containment are considered.

Responsibilities and institutional relationships in economic support for health for all

Chapter V discusses the broad areas of responsibility of different entities involved in health matters. A central concern in formulating national policies on financing health systems based on primary health care is to ensure that resources are used optimally. This requires that responsibility for performance is clearly defined and that adequate mechanisms are established to bring about coordination and effective partnership arrangements.

Key issues discussed and recommendations

Finally, Chapter VI presents the key issues discussed by four working groups during the Fortieth World Health Assembly Technical Discussions. These issues were selected on the basis of the analysis offered in Chapters I–IV of the four broad areas: economic policies for equity in health; financial planning; resources mobilization; and making better use of resources. This chapter also lists the recommendations made by participants in the Technical Discussions with regard to these issues which should be followed up and implemented at the national and international levels.

A glossary of the terms most commonly used in economics is given in Annex 1.

The economic issues influencing health and social development are vast and complex. They are also closely interlinked to the political, social and economic structures and environment of countries. However, there is no doubt that the economic issues are of concern equally to the developed and developing countries, and to the centralized or the market-based decentralized economies and political structures. The composite of issues themselves may be different; for example, in the developed countries where the rising cost of health care is of great concern, high priority may be accorded to issues of cost-containment and cost-sharing, at the same time maintaining levels of quality and effectiveness. On the other hand, in the developing countries, where the provision of at least the essential elements of primary health care to all is the central goal, issues relating to achieving equity through sound planning and efficient and effective use of resources may be paramount.

No single volume can address all the issues adequately or in depth, and thus no attempt has been made to cover the entire spectrum of issues. Moreover, serious deficiency in information related to the availability, distribution and use of financial resources poses further limitations on any analysis offered.

The world economic climate and its implications for health for all

Background

Recent changes in the economic environment have seriously affected the efforts of many countries to implement their strategies for health for all. These economic constraints can at the same time create opportunities for the health sector to play a more dynamic role in dealing with them. The adverse economic situation facing some countries will no doubt continue to challenge policy-makers seeking to achieve a balance between economic and social goals.

Economic and social development are interlinked. The world economic climate has crucial implications for both health and social development. Where there is increasing scarcity of resources, adjustment efforts in macroeconomic policies generally force the social sector to adopt stringent priorities. Efforts that aim to achieve economic growth have to be balanced with those aimed at protecting and promoting human development and pursuing equity-oriented policies. Reduced economic support for the health sector can have serious implications for the effectiveness, efficiency and equity of health services.

Policy-makers face the challenge of identifying the seriousness of these implications and finding new ways to deal with them. New opportunities for improving the quality as well as increasing the quantity of economic support for national health for all strategies need to be explored and be closely linked to the overall development policies of countries.

The ability of countries to invest in health and social development is no doubt influenced to a great extent by trends in their economic development. Similarly, the ability of individuals to pay for their own health services depends on their level of living. Moreover, levels of living are themselves important determinants of health status, as poverty and malnutrition greatly increase vulnerability to disease and are barriers to the attainment of positive health.

There is growing evidence to suggest that despite the economic turbulence, a central issue of concern to all nations of the world is that of quality of life, of which health is an essential ingredient. Many developed and developing countries have demonstrated their political determination to maintain a

The economic development of a country is clearly limited when one out of five children dies before completing one year of life, when a high number of children suffer from stunted growth due to malnutrition, when life-span is shortened by a tenth through disease, or when a significant proportion of the adult population is afflicted by disability and disease.

balance between social and economic development. Health care in the past was considered a privilege for those who could afford to pay, supplemented with charity for the poor; today, health is regarded as a basic human right. This clearly arises out of the recognition that healthy people are essential for economic development.

This chapter briefly discusses the world economic climate, its implications for health and the need for continued political determination for social equity in the face of these trends. It contains four sections. The first summarizes trends in the world economy in the early 1980s as experienced by both the developed and the developing countries and stresses their growing interdependence. The second reviews the effects of the global economy on public sector priorities, especially the extent to which the health sector has been affected by these trends. The third discusses the implications for social development, presenting key arguments for equity and intersectoral action for health. Finally, there is a call for political determination for health for all in times of economic stringency, providing some conclusions for future policy directions for economic support for health care.

Trends in the world economy

The past eight years have been the most turbulent times for the world economy in over half a century. Many of the governments of countries that have achieved independence since 1945 are confronting the most difficult economic challenges that they have ever had to face. The recent changes in the economic environment have seriously affected the ability of governments in developing countries to implement their health programmes and have forced many governments to reassess their spending priorities.

The world's present economic crisis began in 1980 with the onset of the deepest economic recession since 1929. Between 1980 and 1983, per capita production declined in many countries. In the most seriously affected countries of Africa south of the Sahara, western Asia and Latin America, the recession erased the gains made in a decade or more of economic development. In the early 1980s, average living standards fell by 9% in Latin America and by 11% in sub-Saharan Africa. Even the industrialized market economies suffered; the Federal Republic of Germany, the United Kingdom and the USA all recorded a drop in total economic output in one or more of these four years. Unemployment rose to levels that had not been known for half a century.

In 1984 a recovery of global economic growth took place but with wide distortion in the international pattern. Growth in the industrialized countries was nearly 5%, while growth in the developing countries was around 4%. However, growth of nearly 8% in Asia conceals the much lower growth rates of the least developed countries of that continent, and growth in other regions was only 1.5% to 3.1%. It is anticipated that improvement in the relative performance of the developing countries taken as a whole will continue. However, the poorest countries, especially in Africa, are not expected to be in a position to make desired changes in their balance of payments. Faced with a food deficit, they need to continue to import essential goods and services, thus incurring more debts.

The recession has been compounded in many countries by political instability, armed conflicts, natural disasters, and high population growth. In sub-Saharan Africa, the worst drought in 15 years hit many countries in 1982. This devastating drought brought to a head the longer-term adverse trend in food production in this area which has the highest population growth in the world. In the 24 countries most seriously affected by the drought per capita grain production had been falling by 2% per year since 1970.

The economic stagnation which emerged in the early 1980s has been followed by a deepening debt crisis in many countries. The recession in the advanced economies sharply reduced the demand for the goods exported by developing countries. Deprived of part of their anticipated market and thus confronted by a drop in earnings from exports, the heavily-indebted developing countries encountered mounting difficulties in obtaining the foreign currency needed to import drugs, spare parts and replacements for medical equipment, petrol, and other essential materials. The substantial burden of servicing external debts

incurred earlier has further intensified the economic problems of developing countries.

Recently, the sharp drop in oil prices has brought some respite to the balance of payments problems of oil importers. But the problems facing certain oil-producing countries such as Indonesia and Nigeria, where oil represents a high proportion of both export revenue and government revenue, are formidable. Moreover, it has added to the onerous debt-servicing problems that face such countries as Mexico.

These economic problems have forced countries to embark upon economic adjustment programmes which have included efforts to restrain demand for imports and to promote exports. A major tool for achieving these ends has been the devaluation of the local currency in order to make imports more costly and exports more competitive in international markets. Many governments have also attempted to balance their budgets by reducing public expenditure wherever possible. A number of countries have reduced the burden of taxation on firms and individuals in the hope that this would stimulate initiative and private investment. These additional investments in turn were expected to contribute to increased production and thereby lead to greater abundance of both private and public resources.

The world economic climate during the last decade sharply illustrated the economic interdependence of the developed and the developing countries (see Box 1).

Box 1   Economic interdependence

Changes in the pace of economic growth and inflation, protectionism, and shifts in interest and exchange rates in industrialized countries affect developing countries' economic performance through markets for goods and services and through financial markets.

Trade in goods and services

The relative importance of the industrialized countries in world markets for goods has declined moderately in the last fifteen years, but these countries still constitute the major markets for exports and the major suppliers of imports for developing countries. Thus events in industrialized countries have a considerable impact on the prices and volume of goods and services exported by developing countries. A 1% decrease in output in the industrialized economies produces a 2% decrease in commodity prices. Prices of metals and agricultural raw materials, which are used as industrial inputs, more closely reflect cyclical fluctuations in industrial production than do the prices of food and beverages.

Growth in real incomes in industrialized countries also increases the volume of goods imported from developing countries. It is estimated that a 1% increase in the rate of growth in real GNP in industrialized countries results in an increase of about 3.4% in the purchasing power of exports by non-oil-producing developing countries.

Increased protectionism in industrialized countries also has a direct impact on developing countries' export earnings. Protectionism lowers the demand for their exports and thereby depresses prices as well as lowering sales volume. The magnitude of these effects depends as well on the demand in foreign and domestic markets for the goods being traded.

Changes in the prices received for exports and in the volume of foreign sales affect economic growth in developing countries in four ways. Firstly, higher levels of exports raise the overall level of economic activity and thereby increase the rate at which productive capacity is used. Secondly, greater earnings from exports may also promote domestic production by providing foreign exchange with which to purchase scarce imported inputs. The magnitude of this effect depends on a country's dependence on foreign goods and the severity of its foreign exchange constraint. Thirdly, an increase in export earnings alters a developing country's long-term growth prospects by enabling it to raise its rate of investment. Higher export earnings permit larger imports of capital goods; this offers the opportunity of increasing the amount and pace of investment.

(Cont.)

Box 1 (Cont.)

Fourthly, an increase in exports may shift resources from the rest of the economy to the export sectors. This will often accelerate growth because the productivity of the economy is greater in the export sectors than in other parts of the economy. Faster export growth may also encourage other sectors to adopt more productive methods and better management techniques.

Financial markets

The financial system also transmits economic upheavals from country to country. During the 1970s developments in the banking industry in the industrialized countries enabled major banks to lend more to developing countries. At the same time the demand by developing countries for loans increased rapidly because of sizeable balance-of-payments problems caused by two oil shocks. The attractiveness of bank loans derived from their flexibility, convenience and low interest rates. However the use of bank loans to finance developments greatly increased the vulnerability of developing countries to events in world financial markets. Interest payments were due irrespective of the uses to which the original loan had been put, and the amounts due depended on world economic conditions as well.

In the 1980s the disinflationary policies adopted by the industrial countries caused borrowing costs to rise. The change in interest rates was especially large when compared with the prices received by developing countries for their exports. The difference between the real interest rate and the increase in the average prices of exports from developing countries was 18% in 1981-82. These changes in the cost of servicing debts significantly affected the developing economies. For example, the debt service payments of Africa amounted to 27% of export earnings in 1983.

The availability of loans to a developing country also depends on its credit worthiness as perceived by banks. When export earnings decline because of a recession in the industrialized economies, the actual and perceived capacity of a developing country to service its foreign debt is diminished. As a result the impact of a recession is magnified by the consequent abrupt reduction in the availability of external financing and the pressure to repay earlier loans.

Source: Adapted from Goldsborough, D. and Zaidi, I. M. How performance in industrial economies affects developing countries. *Finance and Development*. Vol. 23, No. 4, 1986.

The economic recession and the public health sector

The economic recession on the whole has had a profound effect on domestic priorities and programmes in both the developed and the developing countries. The reduced rate of economic growth has resulted in low growth or even a real decline in government revenues.

Developing countries rely heavily on taxes on imports and export earnings to finance the activities of the public sector. The low-income countries collected a smaller proportion of their Gross National Product in taxes in 1983 than in 1973. For the poorest countries and the newly industrialized, middle-income countries, the decline in the value of international trade between 1979 and 1984 was more than twice as large in percentage terms. Thus the contraction of international trade seriously reduced the collection of government revenues in addition to reducing foreign exchange earnings.

Many governments throughout the world have been forced by the economic events to reduce public expenditure and to consider responses which would have the least damaging impact on social development.

In the market-based industrialized countries, it is clear that there has been a considerable reduction in the rate of growth of expenditure on health services in relation to Gross Domestic Product (GDP). For example, in the OECD countries a rate of growth of 4-5% per year in the percentage of GDP devoted to health services during the period 1965-75 was followed by growth of less than 1% per year. In some of these countries health expenditure has been reduced in real terms over the past two years. Cost-containment has come to be seen as a critical objective. The high cost of supporting the unemployed, either on cash benefits or on special schemes of training or work experience, has led to constraint in other fields of public expenditure. In Europe, cost-sharing has increased considerably, and ceilings have been imposed on public health expenditure and on health expenditure financed by social security. Long-standing problems in the public health sector in the developing countries have no doubt been aggravated by trends in the global and national economy. These countries are faced with the prospect of increasing the utilization of available resources, while at the same time making more adequate resource allocations and reducing inequities in both the sharing of costs and in access to services.

The key question for developing countries is whether per capita expenditure in the health sector has been rising or falling. Very few countries are in a position to answer this question, for a number of reasons. First, public health expenditure may be divided among several government departments, levels of government and statutory agencies (particularly social security funds), and no data may be available for private expenditure by employers, nongovernmental organizations or individuals. Secondly, a special price index would be needed to convert current price figures into constant price figures, particularly for a period with such abrupt changes in terms of trade and devaluations of currencies and, in some cases, deliberate restraint on the salaries of health personnel. Thirdly, even in developed countries there remain problems of defining the health sector in compatible terms.

Because information of this kind is so rarely collected it has been necessary to try to draw conclusions from available data such as those on the percentage of GDP devoted to health services (a narrower concept than the health sector), or even the budget of the ministry of health as a proportion of total central government expenditure.

Only 20 developing countries reported to the United Nations system on national accounts showing relatively recent trends of current public expenditure on health services. Comparing data for 1981 with those for 1983, 10 countries show public health expenditure rising as a proportion of GDP, five show it falling, five others show no change (see Table 1).

Seventeen developing countries, where central government received 90% or more of taxes, reported the percentage of central government expenditure spent on health in 1981 and 1983. In 1983, health secured a higher proportion of national budgets in 10 countries and a lower proportion in 7 compared with 1981 (Table 2).

The trends in public health expenditure, and the widening gap between public expenditures for health in the developed and developing countries are further indicated in Table 3. Per capita expenditure on public health ranges from below US$ 2.00 to well over US$ 500.

Economic crises and the adjustments that result from them exacerbate the "recurrent cost" problem in the health sector in many developing countries. This problem stems from the lack of funds in the public sector with which to operate health facilities and programmes in the manner in which they were designed.

When financial limitations affect public health budgets, the cutbacks in recurrent costs mainly affect the critical inputs required for running services. First cuts are on fuel, vehicles, building and equipment maintenance, supervision, drugs, and other essential inputs. It is easier to cut these than staff salaries. Also lack of foreign exchange for imported drugs, spare or replacement parts and oil has often been serious. As a result of these trends, the effectiveness of staff as well as their morale decreases. Because of lack of quality, facilities are underutilized, especially in the rural areas. The referral and supervision system at the district level has been seriously jeopardized in many countries by cutbacks in recurrent costs, and consequently the delivery of essential health care in rural areas has been curtailed.

The above brief review of the financial problems of public health services should be completed by an analysis of other sources of financing and provision of services. Central governments in many countries rarely contribute more than half of the total funds spent on health activities. Contributions from the state and local governments, nongovernmental organizations (profit-making or non-profit making), communities and

Table 1: Public expenditure on health services as a percentage of gross domestic product, 1977–84

	1977 %	1978 %	1979 %	1980 %	1981 %	1982 %	1983 %	1984 %
Developed countries								
Australia	3.2	3.1	3.0	3.1	3.0	3.0	3.1	3.3
Austria	4.1	4.3	4.3	4.4	4.5	4.5	4.5	—
Finland	4.0	3.9	3.8	3.9	4.0	4.1	4.1	4.4
France	0.4	0.4	0.4	0.5	0.5	0.5	—	—
Federal Republic of Germany	5.7	5.7	5.7	5.9	6.1	5.9	5.8	—
Greece	1.3	1.4	1.5	1.7	1.8	1.9	2.0	2.1
Italy	3.3	3.4	3.6	3.6	3.9	3.9	—	—
Japan	0.4	0.4	0.4	0.4	0.4	0.4	0.4	0.4
Malta	3.4	3.9	3.7	3.9	4.0	4.5	4.5	4.5
Norway	4.1	4.2	4.1	4.0	4.1	4.3	4.4	4.3
Sweden	7.0	7.0	7.0	7.3	7.4	7.5	7.3	—
United States of America	1.1	1.1	1.1	1.1	1.1	1.2	1.2	—
Developing countries								
African Region								
Cameroon	0.7	0.8	0.7	0.6	0.6	0.7	0.8	—
Kenya	1.8	2.1	2.1	2.3	2.3	2.2	2.0	1.9
Lesotho*	1.3	1.2	1.8	2.5	1.8	—	—	—
Mauritania	2.8	2.7	2.4	2.6	2.5	2.4	2.3	2.3
United Republic of Tanzania*	1.8	2.1	1.9	1.7	1.6	1.6	1.5	—
Zimbabwe	1.3	1.6	1.4	1.6	1.6	1.8	1.7	—
Region of the Americas								
Colombia	0.6	0.6	0.7	0.9	0.9	0.9	—	—
Ecuador	0.6	0.7	0.6	0.8	0.9	1.0	1.0	—
Honduras	1.9	1.8	1.8	1.6	1.5	1.4	1.5	—
Panama	1.8	1.6	1.8	1.5	1.5	1.7	1.7	1.7
Peru	1.5	1.5	1.6	1.8	2.0	2.1	2.2	—
Saint Vincent and the Grenadines	4.2	4.7	3.9	3.8	5.0	—	—	—
Venezuela	1.9	2.0	1.6	1.5	1.9	1.9	2.5	2.1
South East Asia Region								
India	0.6	0.6	0.6	0.6	0.6	0.7	0.6	—
Sri Lanka	1.2	1.2	1.1	1.1	1.0	1.0	1.1	1.0
Thailand	0.5	0.5	0.6	0.6	0.7	0.7	0.7	0.8
European Region								
Israel	1.6	1.6	2.0	1.9	1.8	1.8	1.8	—
Eastern Mediterranean Region								
Cyprus	1.3	1.2	1.3	1.5	1.6	1.7	1.7	1.7
Islamic Republic of Iran	1.0	1.0	1.0	1.5	1.3	1.2	1.0	—
Jordan	1.0	0.9	1.0	1.2	1.3	1.3	1.2	1.2
Kuwait	1.4	1.4	1.1	1.4	1.9	2.8	2.5	—
Pakistan	0.7	0.7	0.5	0.4	0.4	0.4	0.5	0.5
Western Pacific Region								
Fiji	2.1	2.1	1.9	1.9	2.1	2.3	—	—
Republic of Korea	—	—	—	0.2	0.2	0.2	0.2	0.2
Tonga	2.9	2.7	2.9	2.6	2.9	3.3	—	—

Notes: * A 'least developed country'.
Source: United Nations National accounts, statistics, main aggregates, and detailed tables, 1982, and computer tapes, New York, United Nations, 1985.

Table 2: Percentage of central government expenditure spent on health in countries where central government received 90% or more of tax revenue, 1977–84

	1977 %	1978 %	1979 %	1980 %	1981 %	1982 %	1983 %	1984 %	1985 %
Developed countries									
Belgium	1.78	1.79	1.86	1.65	1.70	1.65	—	—	
France	14.59	14.83	14.99	15.01	14.72	14.60	—	—	
Greece	8.09	9.89	10.48	10.34	10.54	—	—	—	
Italy	—	7.55	10.47	12.55	10.70	10.64	11.52	11.49	
Luxembourg	2.07	2.27	2.02	2.15	2.37	2.23	2.21	—	
Netherlands	11.79	11.87	11.71	11.68	11.63	11.62	11.29	10.97	
New Zealand	14.98	15.04	15.21	15.17	14.24	13.52	12.65	—	
Developing countries									
African Region									
Kenya	8.16	7.45	7.23	7.83	7.81	7.33	6.96	—	
Lesotho	5.43	—	—	—	—	—	7.18	—	
Liberia	7.89	8.21	6.13	5.20	7.61	7.17	7.27	6.20	
Malawi*	5.40	5.27	5.30	5.53	5.16	5.23	6.77	—	
Mauritius	7.98	8.15	8.04	7.48	6.97	7.10	7.84	8.10	
Swaziland	6.48	4.91	6.29	7.15	5.41	7.12	7.37	—	
Zaïre	4.01	3.94	3.22	2.47	2.61	3.20	—	—	
Region of the Americas									
Chile	6.86	6.85	6.54	7.37	6.54	6.80	5.95	6.18	
Costa Rica	3.31	25.44	25.00	—	—	32.76	22.48	—	
Dominican Republic	8.98	9.43	9.07	9.30	9.70	10.66	10.55	—	
Mexico	4.38	3.97	3.90	2.37	1.86	1.29	1.20	—	
Panama	14.50	15.08	12.15	12.71	13.24	13.14	—	—	
Paraguay	2.73	2.64	3.67	3.59	4.51	3.67	—	—	
Trinidad and Tobago	7.79	6.86	6.36	5.78	5.91	—	—	—	
South East Asia Region									
Burma	5.88	6.73	6.39	5.28	6.09	6.96	—	—	
Maldives*	—	—	5.06	3.46	4.45	5.83	3.80	—	
Sri Lanka	5.95	4.19	5.17	4.88	3.54	3.35	5.12	—	
Thailand	4.69	4.39	4.54	4.09	4.23	4.94	5.11	5.45	
Eastern Mediterranean Region									
Cyprus	5.42	5.92	6.02	6.07	6.73	7.26	6.79	—	
Jordan	3.58	3.71	4.10	—	3.75	3.76	3.63	—	
Kuwait	5.90	5.89	6.25	5.12	4.89	5.38	6.25	6.27	
Oman	2.65	3.17	3.24	2.92	3.04	3.09	3.47	4.13	
Sudan*	1.45	1.71	1.46	1.40	—	1.34	—	—	
Tunisia	7.03	7.27	6.43	7.20	7.65	6.66	—	—	
Western Pacific Region									
Philippines	5.08	4.74	5.54	4.54	5.01	5.28	6.80	—	
Singapore	7.37	8.50	7.01	6.88	7.18	6.39	6.41	—	

Notes * A 'least developed country'.
Source: *IMF Government financial statistics yearbook.* Washington, DC, International Monetary Fund, 1985.

households are important. Over the last decade the proportion of central government expenditures for health care declined in many developing countries while it increased in the developed countries. Data on the allocation of such expenditures from these other sources are neither complete nor reliable. But it seems that the largest part of these resources is spent in the private sector on high-cost, mainly curative, care.

On the demand side there are national and regional variations. Overall, however, the demand is increasing for demographic, epidemiological, economic and sociocultural reasons. The absolute numbers of children and young people in developing countries have been rising. Aging populations and urbanization are increasing the demand for curative services. In many countries, infectious and communicable diseases continue side by side with emerging chronic diseases and health problems related to the environment, behaviour and life-style. An increased awareness of problems through the mass-media and education, especially female education, and improved access to services, are creating a huge potential demand.

Given the lack of uncommitted recurrent budget resources at all levels of the health sector, the feasible scale of reallocation *within* the public health budget will in most countries be too small to allow major, short-term improvements in effectiveness and efficiency. More resources, and the possibility of different sources of finance for health activities, must therefore be sought as a matter of urgency although this may, in some cases, entail a reconsideration of the scope and responsibilities of governments.

The recession and social development

The impact of the economic recession on the industrialized market economies was clearly indicated by the growth of unemployment to an average of around 10%, with one country as high as 21.5%. Hardships are particularly severe in countries that have not yet developed elaborate social security and social welfare schemes and where most families have only one breadwinner. Evidence is accumulating of the different ways in which unemployment

Table 3: **Proportion of public expenditure allocated to health, 1972 and 1983**

Countries	1972 %	1982 %
Low income	6.1	3.0
Industrial market economies	9.9	11.7

Source: World Bank. *World Development Report 1985.* New York, Oxford University Press, 1985.

can damage health. The relationship is complex and multidimensional.

Urban unemployment has also reached high levels in developing countries, nearly all of which lack unemployment insurance. The unemployed join the overcrowded informal sector in an attempt to make some sort of living. Moreover, the unemployed lose their right to use health services financed by social security schemes and the income with which to pay for private services. This adds to demands on the overstrained government health services.

The emphasis on export crops has diverted land from local food production, and the increase in the cost of imports, inflation, high housing costs, the abandonment of food subsidies, as well as high unemployment and underemployment, have made poverty more severe and more widespread in Latin America and the Caribbean. The proportion of babies with low birth weights is on the increase in Brazil and the number of children treated for malnutrition has tripled in Costa Rica. Surveys in six Latin American countries have all indicated increased inequality and poverty.

Poverty has also increased sharply in rural Africa, particularly as a result of the deterioration in terms of trade, increased protectionism, and the recent famine. Certain African countries have suffered outbreaks of yellow fever and cerebrospinal meningitis as well as the effects of the massive displacement of refugees. Surveys from Botswana and Ghana show a clear downward trend in the nutritional status of children, and

in Ethiopia around half the children aged 1–3 are below the standard weight for age. The infant mortality rate rose to 200 or more per 1000 live births in Burkina Faso, Chad, some parts of Ghana, and Mozambique.

At least half of the world's poorest people live in south Asia where the growth of poverty has been greater in the rural than the urban areas. The recession has hit the least developed countries the hardest.

Some national studies on the social impact of the economic deterioration have pointed to increased infant and child mortality, such as in Chile and Costa Rica, deterioration in nutritional status of children, as in Ghana and Zambia, and adverse health effects on adults who have lost employment and income. Of course, the effects of the economic deterioration have been the most evident among the developing countries and within those countries among the poorest people. The health effect of a given total decline in income depends on how the decline is distributed and how the quantity and quality of available health-related services are reduced. Because health determinants are a combination of factors, the health effects of recession and policy readjustments are poorly documented and cannot be easily interpreted.

In general it can be said that the main impact of the recession has been borne by those least able to sustain it, simply because they have neither the political muscle to prevent it nor the economic fat to absorb it. Children have almost certainly suffered most of all in terms

Box 2   Impact of the world recession on the health of children

In 1982, UNICEF initiated a study on the impact of the world recession on the health of children. The findings of that study were reported in a special issue of *World Development* in March 1984. The world economy had undergone two years of what has since been recognized to be the deepest recession in the memory of most living people. The recession persisted for nearly two more years. It was then followed by a deepening debt crisis in much of the developing world outside India and China. In many of the poorest countries, the recovery from the recession has been painfully slow. In a number of African countries, economic growth has not returned to a rate that matches the rate of population growth.

Twelve countries were selected for detailed investigation under the UNICEF study. These countries represented all regions of the world and a wide range of levels of economic and social development. Because the recession was only half-way through when the study was initiated, its effects were presumably not fully manifest. The study found that the greatest suffering seemed to have occurred in Africa. Countries in east and south Asia appeared to weather the first half of the recession with little notable effect on health. A few countries strengthened their programmes to promote health during this period and appeared to have registered gains in health in spite of worsening economic conditions.

The UNICEF study underlined the fact that sensitive indicators of deterioration of health are not available even for small children. The inability to identify changes in mortality and morbidity is in part a consequence of the inability of routinely collected data to reflect changes. The countries studied reported only a limited number of diseases and thus it is possible that important problems were not captured. In addition many of the consequences of economic deprivation are likely to become manifest only after a significant period of time.

A more likely explanation for the lack of dramatic results is that the quantity of care did not decline as markedly as might have been assumed from reductions in the inflation-adjusted budgets of health ministries. Instead, governments reduced non-critical expenditures and allowed staff salaries to decline in purchasing power. Chile, for example, had cut its public outlay for development of new health facilities by nearly 80% between 1969 and 1980. In addition, payments to staff declined in real terms by about 15% over the same period.

Expenditures for supplies over the same period increased by about a quarter. Thus the UNICEF study suggests that considerable short-term adjustment can be made in health budgets in order to maintain levels of

(Cont.)

Box 2 (Cont.)

services. Both public institutions and households appear to be able to reallocate their resources in order to cope with short-term problems of funding. The principal underlying device is to run down equipment, vehicles and buildings by neglecting routine maintenance. These practices may prove costly in the longer term but in the short term allow essential services to be provided on a reduced budget. Such expedients are only workable for a short period of time.

The conclusion that one can draw from the UNICEF study is that the world recession of the early 1980s did not reduce health status significantly but rather delayed further progress in improving the coverage and quality of services. If this failure to increase the supply of health services were to continue for several years, a widening gulf between needs and responses to those needs would become apparent. The challenge then is to resume the process of expanding the supply of effective health care.

Source: UNICEF. *The state of the world's children, 1984.*

of low birth weight, malnutrition, frequency of illness, and poor mental and physical growth.

Very few countries have incorporated their health goals into their adjustment policies, in order to minimize the impact of damage to health and protect high-risk groups most vulnerable to the adverse effects of austerity measures. There is no available evidence that the health sector has suffered from budget cuts more than other social sectors. However, adjustment strategies designed to promote stable economic growth have not taken sufficient account of minimum social needs and equity in the distribution of austerity measures.

Political determination for health for all in times of economic adjustments

The achievement of health goals is determined to a large extent by policies that lie outside the health sector and in particular by policies, whatever their nature, aimed at ensuring universal access to the means of earning an acceptable income. But merely increasing income will not guarantee health. Health authorities will have to display vigilance in identifying aspects of development that can threaten health status and in introducing elements that are essential for health development in their socioeconomic development plans. The links between health and development have been amply demonstrated both by the experiences of developed countries and by the improvement in the quality of

Box 3 **Thailand — Incorporating health improvements in social development**

Thailand, which is in the lower middle-income category (as defined by the World Bank), had an estimated infant mortality rate of 50 per 1000 in 1983 and a life expectancy of 63 years. It had enjoyed an uninterrupted period of economic expansion during the previous 20 years, sustaining an annual average rate of growth between 7% and 8%. National planners, however, noted that "the social gap between the rich and the poor has been increasing" and that "social services such as health and education" had not been developed appropriately and sufficiently "to reach the low income population, especially in the rural areas".

The regional disparities in income and living conditions have remained high. Between 1960 and 1980 the disparity between the poorest region, the north-east, and the richest, the central region, widened. In 1979, the per capita income in the north-east was 40% of the national average and approximately one-sixth of that of the central region. The main pockets of poverty are in the north-east and north, where the proportions of the population below the poverty line have been estimated at 52% and 23% respectively.

The Prime Minister's office organized the Rural Poverty Eradication Programme in 37 provinces throughout the country, assigning to four key ministries (agriculture and cooperatives, education, health, interior) the joint responsibility for formulating and executing the programme under the overall coordination of the National Economic and Social Development Board (NESDB). A key strategy in the programme was job creation for the rural poor to narrow income disparity. At this juncture the NESDB established the Social Development Project to support the Rural Poverty Eradication Programme in problem identification, operational planning and management at the village, subdistrict and district levels. The Social Development Project formulated basic minimum needs and their indicators and elaborated methods for their use as tools for identifying gaps and proposing priority activities at the village level. The Programme was not initially incorporated in the National Social and Economic Development Plan.

When the Fifth National Social and Economic Development Plan was formulated, the Rural Poverty Eradication Programme was incorporated and renamed the Rural Development Programme, the formulation of which was based on experience gained in the application of the basic minimum needs, mentioned above. Examples are "hygienic nutrition to meet physical needs", "adequate shelter and environmental conditions",

(Cont.)

Box 3 (Cont.)

and "development of preschool children". The four key ministries were still jointly responsible for the preparation and implementation of the programme plan, with the continued coordination of the NESDB. Job creation was still its main strategy, but in a wider scope and framework, and a larger proportion of the government budget was allocated to the programme. The Social Development Project was terminated at the beginning of 1985. The Government used outputs of the project, particularly the basic minimum needs and their indicators, as a basis for organizing the National Campaign for the Quality of Life (1985-1986), and they have since been incorporated in the Sixth National Development Plan.

Sources: (1) National Economic and Social Development Board, Thailand. (2) Gunatilleke, G., ed. *Intersectoral linkages and health development*. Geneva, World Health Organization, 1984 (WHO Offset Publication, No. 83).

life in several low-income countries. Ten years ago, the Member States of the World Health Organization unanimously resolved that their main social target should be the attainment by all citizens of the world of a level of health that would permit them to lead a socially and economically productive life. This resolve arose out of a concern to achieve *equity* in health, shrinking the gaps in the health status of people and countries and ensuring equitable distribution of health resources. This called for a concerted political will and response.

The recent evaluation of the national strategies for health for all undertaken by 147 Member States of the World Health Organization has provided evidence that a positive start has been made by countries in their quest for health for all, against a background of deteriorating economic and social conditions (see Annex 2: Evaluation of the strategy for health for all by the year 2000). No doubt, the prevailing and forecasted economic situation will

continue to challenge policy-makers seeking to achieve a balance between economic and social goals.

To protect the poor and vulnerable during the process of adjustment, strategies of adjustment-with-equity are required. Health for all is such a strategy. The reduction of prevailing disparities will require an equitable distribution of health-related resources to bring health care within the reach of vulnerable groups. The causes of disparities in health status can only be removed through intersectoral actions involving the health-related sectors as well as resource allocation policies that give preference to the poor and vulnerable segments of the population, as has been demonstrated by some countries. These aspects were considered during the Technical Discussions on intersectoral action for health at the Thirty-ninth World Health Assembly in 1986. No doubt, the combination of equity, effectiveness and efficiency in the context of economic support emerges as a key

Box 4   Prospects for the health for all strategy

Member States in their reports have reaffirmed the validity of the basic principles of the Strategy. None has mentioned the need to modify the Strategy; for some regions in which substantial progress has been made there has been a call for review and modification of the global indicators.

The Strategy is equally valid for the developing and the developed countries; the latter have adapted it to their particular situation and needs. In the final analysis, national and regional variations will become even more apparent as implementation proceeds.

Three scenarios for the application of the Strategy can be distinguished.

At the top end of the scale are the developed countries and a few developing countries which have made substantial progress in improving health status as well as in making available health services for their populations. These countries are now coping with health problems related to increased life expectancy, to life-styles and to the environment, and their attention is turning to measures to reduce the remaining socioeconomic disparities and to cost-containment policies.

In the middle is perhaps the largest group of countries, those that have made significant progress in establishing a health infrastructure based on primary health care. Their situation is changing, but for the time being they have to deal with both traditional and new health problems. They inevitably find themselves facing new demands with strictly limited resources and at the same time trying to improve the coverage of essential primary health care services. The critical challenge for them is to make maximum use of their resources through strengthened management and improved efficiency. They will also have to mobilize additional internal and external resources.

The countries in the third group – those with the most critically difficult situation – are is still struggling with very high mortality and morbidity, deteriorating socioeconomic conditions and very limited resources to expand the health infrastructure. These countries will require concerted strong support from the international community. They will be called upon to make a serious reappraisal of their national development policies.

Source: Document A39/3 of the Thirty-ninth World Health Assembly, *Evaluation of the Global Strategy for Health for All by the Year 2000, Seventh report on the world health situation*, 1986, paragraphs 476-481.

Box 5 China, Kerala (India), Sri Lanka — The interaction of health and development

In all these areas there is a strong commitment to the goals of equity and concerted efforts to ameliorate the conditions of the disadvantaged and poorer social groups. In all important sectors, the development strategies contain elements aimed at realizing these goals.

The state and public agencies assume an important role in meeting the basic needs of the people. In China, this is the norm, while in Kerala and Sri Lanka, the supply and distribution of certain goods and services essential to basic needs occupy a central place in public policy and are not left to market forces.

Development policies avoid the urban bias common to the strategies of most developing countries in the early phases of their planning. Consequently, resources for the social and economic infrastructure and investment in development are more equitably distributed. The differences in living conditions between rural and urban areas have not been worsened by development. Civic amenities have spread to the rural areas. Sir Lanka, for example, has been able to maintain a rural/urban balance that has limited the internal migration to metropolitan areas.

The political processes are designed such that demands can be formulated and responded to at the community level. In China this is achieved with structures of decentralized decision-making in the communes and lower units. In Kerala and Sri Lanka a highly competitive democratic parliamentary system helps to give forceful expression to community needs and elicit responses from the state.

In economic development programmes, strategies for raising productivity and income in the backward parts of the economy, which contain the poor majority, receive priority. Examples are the diversification of the rural economy, and the increase of productivity and output in agriculture, fisheries, energy, and small-scale industry in China, and the drive for food self-sufficiency through programmes for the improvement of peasant farming and small-scale fisheries in Sri Lanka.

In all three areas high priority is given to education. The strategies pursued have brought education within the reach of the whole school-age population through a system that provides free or heavily subsidized education. Here again, policies are aimed at the equitable distribution of facilities to provide the rural population with access to education. In all three cases, there is a very high level of female participation in the school system. In China, female participation in primary education was (Cont.)

Box 5 (Cont.)

97% in 1982; in Sri Lanka, it was 101%.[a] According to data available for 1978 for Kerala, the rate was 86% as against 55% for the whole of India.

The improvement in the status of women and the removal of forms of discrimination against females as in the case of education have played an important role in enhancing the capacity of the population as a whole for social advancement.

Food security for all segments of the population became an essential objective of public policy. Different policy instruments have been used in each case and include state management of the trade in staple foods (China and Sri Lanka), food rationing with food subsidies (Kerala and Sri Lanka), free food supplements for target groups (Sri Lanka) and land reform to provide scope for food production in small allotments (Kerala).

Note: [a] Percentage enrolled in primary school as a percentage of the age group. It can exceed 100% if some pupils are below or above the country's standard primary school age.
Sources: (1) Gunatilleke, G., ed. *Intersectoral linkages and health development*. Geneva, World Health Organization, 1984 (WHO Offset Publication, No. 83). (2) Halstead, S. B. et al., ed. *Good health at low cost*. New York, Rockefeller Foundation, 1985.

challenge to the national policy-makers. The alleged trade-off between efficiency and equity needs to be recast, to demonstrate efficiency as complementary to equity. Equity represents a highly significant social value, and national political decision-makers cannot isolate themselves or avoid responsibility for decisions that have a profound influence on the level of equity in the assignment of resources and the distribution of health benefits. The making of health policy is a critical task for any society. It is an integral part of the political, economic, legal, and social structure and is but one factor in the decision-making process whereby scarce resources are allocated.

For the policy-makers in the health sector, the implications are obvious. They need to be strong advocates for promoting social priorities in economic adjustment policies. They must mobilize commitment and support from other sectors, especially those closely related to health. And finally, they must develop their capability in defining equitable schemes of financing and of allocation of resources. Their responsibility will be even greater in managing scarce resources more efficiently.

Conclusions

A review of the efforts that have been made to cope with stable or declining resources underlines a serious lack of contingency planning. Little emphasis appears to have been given in the past to planning for variations in economic support for health activities. Instead, governments have approached the management of public finances with considerable optimism about the future availability of funds. Improvements in economic conditions have often been regarded as if they would continue without interruption. At the same time, major reversals such as those that accompanied the oil shocks of the 1970s have been treated as transient.

Recently, officials in the health sector have had to intensify their demands for both government funds and foreign assistance. The failure to mobilize additional funds has been reflected in the *ad hoc* deferral of maintenance for equipment and facilities; failure to supply adequate quantities of drugs, chemicals, medical equipment and other essential supplies; and in some countries delayed payment of staff salaries. These problems and responses are similar to those that have appeared in other sectors. Perhaps the most important lesson to arise from the present economic crisis is that more thorough financial planning is needed than has been practised in the recent past by public sector agencies. In particular, these experiences suggest a need to devise methods for financing public services that are less vulnerable to short-term economic fluctuations, and a need to develop plans for coping effectively with financial problems when they arise.

Progress towards health for all is not furthered by overambitious policies that cannot be financed and that fall into disarray when economic development does not progress at the anticipated rate. More modest plans that can be sustained are more likely to reach the desired goals. If sacrifices have to be made in response to an economic crisis, the main aim should be to protect the poor and vulnerable. It should be remembered that good health is one of the purposes of economic development and that, in the long run, health promotes economic development.

External economic factors must not be allowed to become the scapegoat for underachievement in the health sector. There is much that the health sector itself can do to make better use of available resources and, by sound financial planning and stringent managerial procedures, reduce waste and increase efficiency. The health sector also needs to create stronger partnerships with other sectors of development, with nongovernmental organizations and the private sector, and to draw upon the support of local communities by involving them in all its activities at the local level.

Chapter II

Planning and managing the finances

Background

The elaboration of a well defined national plan of action, including a financial master plan, is an essential part of the strategy for attaining health for all. The sources of finance for the implementation of the plan of action differ widely among countries according to the particular circumstances. The need for a national framework to deal with the implementation of strategies and plans of action or their readjustment is especially evident in a period of economic austerity. The recession and the succeeding debt crisis of the 1980s have revealed that the arrangements now being used to finance health for all strategies are inadequate in many developing countries.

Chapter I discussed the impact of the world economic climate on the public sector, especially the public health sector. The quantity of resources being devoted to health programmes is not expanding as rapidly as was anticipated a few years ago. Some of the poorest countries have relied on continued and even expanded concessionary assistance from others to finance the development of facilities and their operation and maintenance. It is evident that the developed economies cannot be relied upon to meet these needs, particularly on a long-term basis.

The Global Strategy for Health for All called upon Ministers of Health "to present to their governments a master plan for the use of all financial and material resources". In January 1986, the Executive Board of WHO, noting

the subject for the Technical Discussions to be held during the Fortieth World Health Assembly, urged "those Member States which have not already done so:

a) to develop further their national strategies for health for all by the year 2000 by producing costed plans for health services and health-related activities;

b) to investigate all possible sources of finance, including the deployment of existing resources;

c) to ensure that the plans can realistically be contained within the resources expected to be available."[1]

This chapter focuses on improved financial planning and management as a way of increasing the effectiveness of available resources and of reducing the vulnerability of the sector to external economic events. The chapter contains five sections. The first discusses the elaboration of a financial master plan as a device for determining the financial feasibility of implementing strategies for health for all. The second sets out different possible ways of closing the resource gaps. The third considers the need to improve budgeting and, in particular, to introduce programme budgeting in order to improve budget preparation and control over the use of resources. The fourth examines changes in accounting practices that would strengthen the management of the

---

[1] Resolution EB77.R11.

day-to-day operations of the sector. The fifth discusses choices of sources of revenue to try to ensure the stability of financing arrangements. Finally, the main conclusions of this analysis and their implications for national policy decisions are summarized.

Financial master plan

The financial implications of declared health policies need to be estimated. National plans of action for health for all that are found to be financially unfeasible should be modified, while still ensuring that the compromises and changes are consistent with national health policies. National health plans typically elaborate the investments in manpower, facilities, equipment and training that would be required in order to achieve, by a prescribed date, targeted levels of coverage or of access to services. Often the implications of these investments for recurrent outlays are not assessed systematically. Estimates of the future costs of paying staff, maintaining buildings and equipment, providing drugs and supplies, and replacing obsolete and worn out capital items are needed in order to ensure that funds are adequately budgeted. Moreover, there are often competing commitments and promises to provide new hospitals, rebuild hospitals or develop specialized units of which the full long-term financial implications have not been calculated. While national health plans specify the expansion of capital and human investments required, they rarely include calculations of the recurrent budgets needed to make full use of these investments. Instead, the commitments of governments to

provide specified services have been conveniently interpreted as implying a pledge to provide the corresponding funds as well.

The events of the past few years have revealed that the financial feasibility of national health plans needs to be appraised in much greater detail. In many countries national health plans have been found to be impossible to fund, and hence to implement. Commitments to provide services often could not be honoured with the financial resources available from government budgets and from such other measures as governments have contrived to generate funds for the health sector. The shortfall in funding has manifested itself in delayed implementation of policies to provide everyone with reasonable access to services, and in a compromised quality of care as a result of inadequate provision of vaccines, drugs, supplies, staff, transport, and maintenance of existing facilities. Hence, well-intentioned commitments to provide universal access to essential health services remain to be fulfilled. In order to meet these pledges, improved financial planning and management and better mechanisms for mobilizing funds are needed.

The preparation of a *financial master plan* is an essential step towards ensuring that health policies that are reflected in a national plan of action to achieve health for all can be successfully implemented. Such plans would anticipate the capital and recurrent costs of implementing the countrywide programmes included in the proposed plan and would identify sources of funds to meet these requirements. The process seeks only to identify the boundaries within which a health plan could be implemented. Hence, a master plan may be based on fairly rough estimates of the costs of the plan and compared with modest projections of the growth of national income, tax revenues and other existing sources of finance used to support the health sector.

The first essential step is to calculate how the health plans have been financed over recent years, including the contribution of the private sector. The second step is to estimate the costs of meeting proclaimed health goals and to distribute these costs over a period of time between the initiation of the plan and the year 2000. This projection of capital and recurrent costs would then be compared with the revenues likely to become available from existing sources of finance. The third step is to explore all possible further sources of finance. This is discussed further in Chapter III. The final step is to reconcile planned expenditure with the revenue both from existing and further sources of finance. Any gap must be eliminated – if necessary by recasting planned expenditure so that it fits the available revenue by, for example, finding efficiency savings, a less costly manpower mix, or using more appropriate technology.

Experience with financial planning

A few countries have developed full financial master plans. Box 6 gives some brief examples.

Closing the resource gap

While the countries mentioned in Box 6 have found it feasible to finance their health plans, many others will find a gap between the resources likely to be available from all possible sources and their first draft of a costed plan. Several options for achieving financial feasibility need to be considered. First, the period over which some parts of the policy are to be implemented may be extended. By taking a longer time to achieve the goals, the extra funds required each year for capital investments and consequential recurrent costs can be reduced. Analysis may also reveal that a greater coverage could be obtained more rapidly by more careful scheduling of expansion. The cost per person will generally be highest where population densities are lowest and social infrastructure is least developed. Thus coverage can often be accelerated by phasing the expansion, starting with the most populated areas. However, considerations of equity and of absolute need may argue for an implementation strategy that maximizes the impact of the government's health activities rather than coverage.

Secondly, the gap between needs and resources may be closed by lowering the goals for the content or extension of services. The gains from reductions in the content of health care are likely to be small since deleting a particular service will significantly affect costs only if it permits the system to operate without a category of staff or a major item of equipment. Targeting the most vulnerable group is also a way to reduce the gap.

Box 6 **Some examples of financial master plans**

Costa Rica plans to achieve health for all by the year 1990. Despite an average income per head of US$ 1334, the expectation of life at birth exceeds 73 years and the infant mortality rate is 18 per 1000. The hospital system is already well developed and the use of beds is steadily adjusting to the aging population. One of the main thrusts of policy since 1980 has been to integrate the mainly curative services provided by Social Security with the preventive services provided by the Ministry of Health. In 1985, 65% of the population were serviced by integrated primary health care units: this will rise to 100% by the year 2000. From 1988 it is planned that each member of the population will be able to choose a general practitioner who will provide a 24-hour service as a member of a multidisciplinary team. Services are to be decentralized, local participation increased and intersectoral coordination is to be strengthened. Piped water is to be extended from 88% of the rural population to 100%. The plan envisages an increase of 79% in the current cost of the preventive service provided by the Ministry of Health and of 45% in the mainly curative services provided by Social Security. Within the latter, expenditure on out-of-hospital services is to grow faster than expenditure on hospital services. The percentage of GNP devoted to health services is to fall from 7.3% in 1987 to 6.7% in 1990 mainly as a result of a decline in capital construction.

The *Netherlands* plan is based on a policy document submitted to parliament in 1986 which sets out national policies, targets and strategies up to the year 2000. The plan envisages an annual growth of health expenditure of 1.2% in response to the changing morbidity pattern, particularly caused by the aging population. The growth rates for the different parts of the health care system are shown below.

	Expenditure in 1986	Annual growth rate
	(Guilder millions)	
Administration	2.5	0.5
Specialist care	1.8	0.5
Drugs	3.7	0.8
Hospital care	20.5	1.3
Collective preventive care	0.8	1.5
Primary health care	5.9	1.9

The share of health care in the GNP is expected to decrease from 8.3% in 1986 to 7.8% in the year 2000.

(Cont.)

Box 6 (Cont.)

The plan in *Sweden* is based on an Act which came into force on 1 January 1983. The policy is to secure good health and health care on equal terms for the entire population. The plan takes account of the growth in the elderly population and provides for effective collaboration between the medical and social sectors. A larger proportion of resources is to be devoted to the prevention of disease and injury, to primary health care, to care in the home and small institutions, and improving the environment. County hospital beds for secondary and tertiary care are to be cut by 28% and psychiatric beds by 50%. Despite these reductions, the cost of the health care system is planned to continue to rise, although at a far more moderate rate than in previous decades. Health care represented 7.8% of Sweden's GNP in 1983, and will reach 8.0% in the year 2000. Secondary and tertiary care (other than psychiatric) as a share of the total health budget will drop from the 1983 figure of 60% to 48% in the year 2000; psychiatric care will fall from 17% to 13% and primary care will rise from 23% to 39% of the total.

Zimbabwe plans to complete the coverage of the population by rural health centres supported by upgraded and new district hospitals by the year 2000. Among the targets are the reduction of infant mortality to less than 50 per 1000 live births, childhood mortality to less than 20 per 1000 and maternal mortality to 100 per 100 000 with 90% of deliveries attended by trained personnel. The percentage of children immunized is to be raised to 80%. The financial plan was built up by costing capital developments and their recurrent costs and manpower training requirements, and costing the plan of action so as to add any further expenditures not included in the main programme. About 90% of the additional expenditure required is for primary health care. Health sector spending is planned to grow by 80% by the year 2000 financed by the estimated growth in tax revenue, with the crucial addition of a new health insurance scheme.

Source: Detailed case studies in financing health development – options, experiences and experiments. Unpublished WHO document, HSC/87.1, 1987.

A third option for reducing the gap between demands for resources and their availability is to reduce the accessibility of care. This option implies either locating facilities further apart or constructing and operating smaller facilities. These reductions in services may increase the time required for travel and waiting for at least some consumers of the health services and thereby discourage their use. Whether this will have a serious effect on the health of the people will depend on which demands are left unsatisfied.

A fourth alternative for closing the gap is to change the mix of manpower and use staff with less training for primary health care. A fifth possibility is to reduce the ratio of staff working in primary health care to the population so as to be able to extend coverage at a faster rate. This may require a tighter definition of the tasks to be performed. Plans vary widely in their manpower components. For example, one country in sub-Saharan Africa plans to provide primary health care with 6 paid staff per 1000 population and another with 3 paid staff per 1000. Both plans envisage providing all the eight essential elements of primary health care.

The ultimate objective of a financial master plan is to establish mutual consistency of the health goals and funding policies. By establishing the financial feasibility of an overall policy for the sector, governments may avoid inadvertently providing care in a manner that is inequitable and unsustainable.

Programme budgeting

A comprehensive programme to improve financial management includes strengthening of the budget function in order to increase the efficiency and effectiveness of health care. Measures to increase the efficiency of other public sector programmes would also be useful, but health authorities have little direct influence over them. While a financial master plan will help to establish whether a policy can be implemented, annual budgets identifying the particular investments and activities that require financial support during the year are required for the implementation of programmes. The budgeting system should stress the links between programme objectives and the use of resources and the relationships between capital expenditure and recurrent costs.

In order to introduce programme budgeting, concrete programme objectives must first be specified. Detailed plans for achieving those objectives can then be devised, and finally the expected accomplishments and the detailed costs of these plans estimated. During the implementation of the programme objectives, accomplishments and costs should be carefully monitored to ensure that plans are realized and any necessary modifications made.

This approach to budget formulation and expenditure control emphasizes achievements rather than resource inputs. It departs from traditional public sector budgeting and accounting in two important respects. First, it stresses the preparation of budgets and summary, of expenditures by objective ("product" or "outcome") rather than by item of expenditure. Thus the primary breakdown of the accounting system is into categories such as "supply of drinking-water to homes" or "care of pregnant women", rather than "pipes", "vehicles", or "drugs". Secondly, the accounting system associated with programme budgeting enables managers to monitor the relationship between the costs and the achievement of a particular objective. By recording expenditures according to the purpose for which they are to be used, managers can oversee the efficiency of a programme rather than merely the extent of its compliance with budget authorizations.

Systems of budgeting that stress the relationship of expenditure to activities may be further elaborated in order to produce estimates of the costs incurred by each management unit in meeting defined objectives. The performance of individual management units and providers of services may then be evaluated. For example, the quantity of drugs employed by each rural dispensary in the treatment of a case of malaria might be determined and analysed. Dispensaries reporting exceptionally high or exceptionally low rates of drug use could then be followed up by supervisors. The effective use of budgeting and cost-accounting to strengthen management requires the collection of information about the activities as well as the finances of the sector. In addition, management applications require that information on health activities be collected and assigned to organizational units that have sufficient autonomy and authority to be held accountable for both their performance and for their use of resources.

Improving financial accounting

Conventional governmental accounting systems provide a basis for budgeting and help to ensure that expenditures have been sanctioned, and to guard against the unauthorized use of funds. These purposes may be met by simply recording all spending under the

headings used in the government's budget document. However, in order to determine the cost of providing a particular product or service, additional information is needed. Not only must outlays be associated with programme outputs but expenditure must be adjusted to ensure that the quantity of resources used is distinguished from quantities purchased. Resources that are totally consumed during the period in which they were purchased (the services of a health worker, for example) may be charged directly to costs. However, expenditures that are expected to contribute to output over several reporting periods (such as a hospital bed, a vehicle, or a stock of drugs) should be recorded separately and distributed over the activities or periods for which they are inputs. In addition, the replenishment of stocks and the withdrawal of goods from inventories for use should be distinguished. The accounts should also identify the purposes for which items were withdrawn.

A well conceived accounting system will permit managers to determine the full cost of carrying out an activity or meeting an objective. They may then compare the costs experienced over time, at various locations and under different supervisors, in order to identify good and bad management of resources.

Coordinating revenue and expenditure

The current economic crisis has demonstrated that reliance on periodic appropriations from governments for all or even a substantial part of the funding of health programmes places the sector at the mercy of events beyond its, and even national government's, control. Thus there is a need to plan ways of obtaining funds that, as far as possible, avoid these risks.

In planning how funds are to be obtained, several principles and distinctions need to be kept in mind. First, interruptions in the flow of funds to an agency can have a catastrophic effect not only on its operations over the short term but also on its capacity to perform in the future. The lack of funds will normally be accommodated by neglecting the expenditures that may be delayed with the fewest legal or political consequences. Formal legal obligations to repay foreign and private domestic debts, or to pay staff salaries, are likely to be honoured, while expenditure needed to service vehicles or maintain buildings is likely to be deferred. A deferral of maintenance and a reduction in service quality are the most common responses to financial short falls.

Authorities in hospitals and clinics delay the maintenance of buildings and equipment in order to save money. Water supply authorities often reduce the amount of the chemicals used to clarify and disinfect drinking water while continuing to pay salaries and electricity charges so that the production and distribution of water is not interrupted. Most agencies continue to provide services although the service may no longer be effective or safe.

In the long term such efforts to cope with financial problems are likely to

destroy public confidence in a service, to erode the morale of staff, and to undermine the traditions of health care institutions. The deterioration of facilities and reductions in service quality are eventually recognized by the clients and customers. Perhaps more seriously, the staff of the service or agency typically suffer a loss of professional confidence and self-esteem as service quality and customer satisfaction deteriorate. This loss often results in a permanent reduction of professionalism and commitment to technical standards. Moreover, in cases where salaries cannot be paid or where long periods elapse with no adjustment in salaries to compensate for increases in living costs, trained staff are likely to leave the service, thereby wasting earlier investments in their training.

In many of the subsectors related to health the costs of inadequate operation and maintenance can be very high. For example, failure to lubricate the bearings on a water pump may result in irreparable damage to the shaft of the pump; thus, a saving of less than a dollar may eventually force the agency to replace an item of equipment costing thousands of dollars. Similarly, a failure to paint buildings or to repair leaking roofs may irreparably damage the structures.

In a long-term financial plan, sources of funds, their likely yield, and their adequacy for meeting the future needs of a programme should be determined. As indicated above, a reliance on periodic appropriations from legislative bodies is an unsatisfactory method of meeting these needs. Competing public sector priorities and short-term financial and economic crises are likely to result, from time to time, in inadequate allocations to the health sector. These reductions may not be so much a reflection of the priorities of governments as the legal and diplomatic options available to them. For example, countries would be likely to lose their access to international credit if they default on their external debts. While reducing the scale of a domestic programme may be very painful, isolation from foreign suppliers would be catastrophic, especially for smaller countries that are dependent on imports and exports.

The methods used to secure funds should be coordinated with the requirements for financing. Often governments have found it more expedient to have services, which should be their direct responsibility, paid for by foreign or domestic lenders, and to pay their external debt obligations instead. The authorities of water supply services have negotiated agreements with governments whereby the cost of providing free services to the poor through public standpipes is financed by a one-time contribution to the capital development programmes of water authorities. The servicing of the debt arising from the contribution then becomes the direct responsibility of governments rather than an obligation of the water authorities, which has to be met from periodic appropriations from the government. Whenever a practical justification can be found, health agencies should minimize their obligations to repay long-term debts.

A second measure for managing the financial requirements of an agency is to link generation of revenue to the delivery of services. Even countries that are not faced with the problems of external debt or a sluggish domestic economy may face problems in paying for public services because inflation and increasing demand outstrip the yield of the taxes or fees dedicated to financing the service. Local governments face this problem most frequently; because higher levels of government establish tax rates and often reassess the value of properties on which tax liabilities are calculated as well, local authorities have little control over the yield of their tax system. As a result, revenues may remain constant as costs rise because of inflation, creating a financial crisis.

Where the revision of fees must be approved by the political authorities, similar problems confront authorities that provide services on a fee basis. For example, attempts to finance water and sewerage services from fees have frequently been frustrated by governments' refusal to approve rate increases to compensate for inflation. Several countries have authorized the periodic recalculation of fees to reflect changes in the prices of inputs.

A good financial plan seeks to meet the need for additional funds by relying on measures that may be expected to expand in parallel with a programme's expenditures. The general sales tax and the value added tax, for example, produce revenues that keep pace roughly with both inflation and the growth in incomes, since these taxes are calculated on the basis of the market values of goods and services. A social security contribution related to earnings keeps pace with the growth of earnings. Such taxes and contributions are therefore ideal for financing services that are likely to need to grow with incomes. User charges are attractive ways of financing services whose cost depends very much on the volume of services demanded. On the other hand, services whose costs are almost unrelated to the rate of use may be paid for with taxes or fees that provide a stable revenue. Sewerage provides an example. The bulk of the cost of waterborne sewerage is the initial capital investment. This investment is usually financed on terms and at prices established for the entire life of the system. Financing these costs from a betterment levy or addition to the real property tax is therefore practical since the financial requirements are known with considerable precision decades in advance. The additional costs of repairs, energy, labour, and chemicals are relatively modest. These recurrent operating costs can be met by a surcharge on the water charge or from a separate assessment.

Several important distinctions need to be borne in mind in examining the costs that must be financed and how they might best be met. First, are the costs fixed for long periods? Costs incurred in constructing facilities, training staff, or developing a programme may vary little. If the annual outlay is then known with confidence many years in advance, the means of finance simply needs to be reliable and does not need to expand with inflation or economic growth. The general property tax is a good example of such a revenue device.

Second, are the costs of the programme likely to increase in a systematic manner over time? If the answer is yes,

then a financing mechanism that grows for similar underlying reasons is desirable. For example, a rural health care programme has costs that are likely to expand roughly in step with inflation and the growth of the population. This pattern of costs reflects the dominance of salaries, drugs and supplies in the overall costs of dispensaries. Therefore, the subsector should have a financing mechanism that is responsive to these underlying forces. A tax on income or the value of production would meet this requirement.

Third, are costs closely linked to choices made by households? The quantity of water used varies widely among households, by season and by income class. Charges based on the volume demanded provide a means of coordinating revenues and costs.

Conclusions

The planners' task is essentially to develop options for political decision-making. Deciding on which mechanisms will be used to finance the health plan is inevitably a political process. Many of the issues are highly sensitive and will require discussion between ministers of health, health-related sectors and those responsible for national planning and finance, with representatives of employers and employees and other organizations, and will finally need the approval of the president or cabinet as a whole. Ministers need to encourage their planning staff to engage in creative thinking, even if some of the options presented prove to be politically unacceptable.

Good financial planning and management are essential to the implemention of national health for all policies and strategies. The total financial requirements implied by the strategies have to be compared with the expected flow of resources. Mechanisms for adjusting either the programmes to be implemented or the financing of the plan are complex. A continuous dialogue is therefore required between staff at many levels of the health system, socioeconomic development planners, the community, the private sector, and nongovernmental organizations. The planning process is an essential tool in policy-making and in realizing political commitments to shift to a more equitable allocation, distribution and utilization of health resources.

The effectiveness of the planning process depends on the extent to which it results in a more efficient and equitable use of resources. Decisions are determined by various interacting factors such as internal political commitment, external influences, nongovernmental initiatives, and government planning processes. Throughout the various stages from policy formulation to the practical implementation of a designed plan, political commitment needs to be steadily reaffirmed.

Planners and managers have to provide relevant information and propose options for political decision-makers so as to make the government's health for all policy a coherent whole, reflecting the critical social value of equity. A close relationship between planners and decision-makers, and a clear understanding and recognition of their respective roles, are prerequisites for successful planning.

Chapter III

Mobilizing resources

Background

In Chapter II, it was stressed that preparation of a financial master plan and improved financial management can reduce the vulnerability of a nation's health plan to macroeconomic problems and to shifts in political priorities. Increases in coverage, and the maintenance and improvement of content and quality, however, will in many cases require that additional resources be committed to health programmes. The amounts of money that can be allocated to health programmes by government will depend not only on health needs but on the competing priorities within the country, as well as its economic resources. Even the developed countries, faced with escalating costs of health care, the aging of their population and the questionable value and effectiveness of some technologies, are reassessing their strategies to provide adequate health care to all.

This chapter presents and evaluates the options that are available to governments in order to mobilize resources for health. It first outlines the issues and criteria that should be considered in choosing a financial

strategy. It then reviews different options for mobilizing resources, including community financing, discussing their potential for financing health for all.

Criteria for choosing a financing strategy

Strategies for financing health for all will reflect the various characteristics of national economies. Where the government is predominant in the production and allocation of goods and services, and where the economy is monetized, the level and composition of health sector financing are both identifiable and, in principle, easily controllable. Where, on the other hand, there are multiple agencies of government, together with important private and nongovernmental sectors, the role of the public sector is more complex. Government financing strategies will affect not only publicly provided services, but also those of the private sector and nongovernmental organizations. Harmonization among the different agencies contributing to health for all will necessitate the following criteria being considered not only for government programmes, but

---

Box 7   Criteria for choosing a financing strategy

Equity
Adequacy
Reliability
Impact on supply
Impact on demand
Intersectoral linkages
Administrative feasibility

for each quasi-independent health subsector individually. Regulation and coordination, often with the ministry of health enjoying only limited statutory authority, become essential additions to service provision.

Equity

Any strategy for mobilizing resources for health for all must be concerned with equity; this implies that policy-makers must be concerned not only with who gains from health programmes but also with who pays for them. Government-financed and operated programmes affect the distribution of services and benefits among individuals. Plans for providing public services that are overambitious cannot be fully implemented and hence some people may be denied access to them, which is inequitable.

The issue of equity also arises in connection with the methods used to obtain inputs to public programmes. Government revenues are obtained ultimately from individuals and households through various forms of taxation, such as taxes on income, business, production (including the value added tax), land, buildings, vehicles, animals and personal property; fees and licences imposed on professions and businesses; import and export duties; and excise taxes on entertainment and luxury goods.

Most taxes affect some groups more than others and therefore redistribute after-tax incomes. In considering the impact of a tax on the distribution of income, one must recognize that many taxes can be shifted from the person legally required to pay it to customers, workers, tenants of land, or suppliers of

raw materials. Such shifting of taxes may then result in a very different impact on the distribution of economic welfare than was originally intended.

The developing countries rely most heavily on taxes on imports and exports and on sales because these taxes are easy and inexpensive to administer. As prices are set by international markets, export duties reduce prices paid to producers, regardless of who is legally responsible for making the payment to the government. Since basic, raw commodities – agricultural goods, timber, ore, fish, and so on – are the principal exports of most developing countries, the burden of financing government services falls mostly on farmers, timber harvesters, mine operators and fishermen. Taxes on imports are also an important source of government revenue in many developing countries. These taxes affect prices paid by consumers for foreign manufactured goods, and thus fall most heavily on people who spend a large share of their incomes on these imports.

Inflated exchange rates also produce revenue for governments by, in effect, taxing exports. Producers of export goods receive less local currency from their sales, and importers obtain more foreign goods per unit of local currency. This relatively inconspicuous form of taxation falls especially hard on the rural poor.

Taxes on income and wealth (real estate or personal property) are not so readily shifted on to other people and therefore permit governments to impose taxes in a less capricious and more equitable manner, but such taxes are difficult to administer in developing countries and may also be easily evaded. Social security contributions, on the other hand, which take a percentage of earnings (often subject to a maximum income beyond which the "tax" is not levied) are easier to administer because: (a) the task of collection falls on employers, and (b) there are no complicated allowances varying between individuals which exempt the first part of income from taxation. Such taxes can, however, only be readily collected from those with regular jobs working for large employers. In developing countries these are generally a minority of the working population, but their incomes are on average higher than those in the informal sector or in subsistence agriculture. Social security contributions are widely used to finance health services in developed countries and are often retained as a source of income when the same rights to services are extended to the whole population by a national health service. They are also a major source of income for the health sector in some developing countries – particularly in Latin America – often contributing more revenue than taxes.

In the least developed countries, governments rely heavily on indirect taxes, which fall especially heavily on those who must spend a large share of their income on taxable goods. Thus the poor are usually adversely affected. For this reason, taxes may be an inequitable way of raising funds to finance national strategies for health for all. This is of particular importance where services are unevenly distributed. Those without access to

services may be paying taxes to finance services enjoyed primarily by the urban population.

Adequacy

The second issue in considering financial strategies is whether the device for producing revenue will yield enough money to meet the needs. This issue of adequacy arises frequently in the least developed countries where the taxes that are administratively feasible often do not produce enough revenue to finance essential government services. If the taxes on goods are raised too much, the underlying activities may become unrewarding. The yield from the tax will then vanish. For example, in one West African country high taxes on exports of cocoa made production unprofitable for farmers, who then stopped cultivating it. The country lost its share of the international cocoa market.

The question of the adequacy of revenue-raising systems also arises as the revenue needs of a health programme develop and mature. A revenue plan that is serviceable now may be inadequate a few years hence unless its methods of revenue generation produce a corresponding growth in funds. In recent years, this problem has emerged primarily because inflation has escalated costs and the yield of taxes has not grown with inflation. Social security taxes, payroll levies, excises on farm commodities, proceeds of lotteries and taxes on tobacco, alcohol, and entertainments have been dedicated to financing health activities in some countries. These revenue sources differ widely in their responsiveness to such factors as inflation, population growth, and social development. Some may be inadequate solutions to the provision of sustained financial support for health services.

Reliability

The revenues produced by a tax, or fee, or foreign assistance may vary considerably with economic conditions. For example, if the revenue system used to support health services is based largely on taxes on the export of a commodity used in industrial production, then its yield is likely to rise and fall with economic conditions in industrialized countries. The funds available to pay for salaries, drugs, spare parts and maintenance of existing vehicles and facilities may become severely inadequate during a recession. (This sequence of events was encountered by a number of developing countries in the early 1980s.) Reliability is likely to be a particularly serious problem if funds are obtained from general government revenues by periodic legislative appropriation.

Impact on supply

Revenue systems produce incentives which may influence the decisions and attitudes of both managers and providers of health services. The principal mechanism for transmitting incentives from the revenue system to the health care institution is the formula used in determining its budget. For example, if additional funds are provided to institutions with a heavy responsibility for specialized problems or endemic diseases, the staff is likely to be more vigilant in identifying these problems. The incentives inherent in a revenue and budgeting system may be harnessed to promote desirable health outcomes. This requires that the incentive mechanisms are fully

recognized and understood, and that the organization of and responsibility for services and for the management of resources be designed to take advantage of these effects. Even if institutions are thoroughly committed to the public interest, the incentives need to be scrutinized to ensure that they confirm and reward desirable behaviour.

Impact on demand

Revenue mechanisms also affect the use of services by the public. User charges provide a direct link between the use of services and the financing of the system. This link clearly discourages the utilization of services. The magnitude of this effect clearly depends upon the wealth and income of the potential user of services and on his/her illness. If consumers are well informed, the effect will be to focus scarce resources on the most serious problems: however, most consumers are unable to make such distinctions in assessing their health care requirements.

A large part of the cost of utilizing health care facilities is borne by households in the form of travel expenses, and earnings lost while seeking care. Often several family members accompany seriously ill people to the hospital or clinic, thereby increasing the cost of health care to the family. The magnitude of these costs depends on proximity to health care facilities, the number of referral steps needed to obtain drugs or competent care, the season, and the age and sex of the patient.

The impact of policies on the siting of health care facilities, the range of services offered at each site and the referral of patients should be recognized. These factors affect both the costs of supplying services and the burden on households using the health care system.

Intersectoral linkages

Primary health care includes not only personal medical services but also such activities as health education, water supply, sanitation, nutrition, and vector control. Several of these services are provided jointly with services that are not directly under the responsibility of the health sector. For example, some health education is provided concurrently with primary education, and water for drinking and washing is often supplied together with water for industrial processes, landscape gardening and fire-fighting. Health sector financing strategies should stimulate intersectoral action in favour of health, even though responsibility is not assumed for activities in which health is a joint output.

Administrative feasibility

The successful introduction and operation of any mechanism for generating revenues require that practical methods be available for assessing the obligations of each person, enforcing payment and safeguarding the revenues collected. These requirements are most demanding in countries where the formal bureaucracy and traditions of compliance with tax laws are not highly developed. Tax compliance depends frequently on recognition by the people that the burden of paying for government and for specific programmes is fairly distributed. In addition, the public generally accepts taxes more readily if they are

convinced that they are being administered conscientiously. User charges can be more acceptable than taxes based upon income, wealth or economic activity, since user charges are linked to the benefits gained from a programme. Social security contributions may be more acceptable than taxes because people know what they are paying for.

If local officials are not highly accountable to the community or carefully supervised, funds may be diverted to personal use and collections may be unevenly enforced. The administration of a revenue system is less subject to abuse if the scope and quality of services available locally depend on the funds collected. However, tax-payers and users may refuse to make payments if they suspect that others are avoiding payment, of if services are not available.

Options for financing strategies for health for all

Many options for financing services are now being widely considered. They may be grouped into five major categories. First, governments may pay for health care from *public revenues.* These revenues are obtained from some combination of income taxes, sales taxes, export levies, import duties, licence fees, foreign assistance, and so on. Second, a variety of *insurance* schemes for the sharing of risks is possible. Compulsory and voluntary shares are discussed separately. Third, schemes of *community financing* may be developed. Fourth, consumers may

> ### Box 8   Options for further financing
>
> - Attract more tax revenue, possibly from earmarked taxes.
> - Attract more external cooperation.
> - Introduce or extend compulsory health insurance.
> - Require employers to provide defined services.
> - Introduce charges or raise charges for government services.
> - Encourage fund-raising by nongovernmental organizations.
> - Stimulate community financing and voluntary health insurance.
> - Make savings through a more efficient use of resources.
> - Reorient priorities within existing services, or select less costly methods of service delivery.

be required to pay *user charges* to meet part of the cost of the health services they use. A large number of variants of these themes have been devised, each of which has distinctive economic, financial or administrative attributes. Finally, the roles of *nongovernmental organizations* and *external cooperation* are considered.

Direct government financing

Direct government financing of health activities is perhaps the most widespread approach to health financing in the developing world. Governments either provide periodic allocations from general government revenues or assign the proceeds of a designated tax to the health sector, or both.

Public revenues are obtained from various sources and then generally are added together. Thus the source of financing for a particular public programme cannot be identified. However, in some cases, governments dedicate the proceeds of a particular

tax instrument to the health sector. A dedicated tax provides the sector with a relatively reliable source of income whose likely yield can be estimated several years in advance. Some governments (especially in Latin America) have chosen to allocate the proceeds of taxes on tobacco, alcohol, gambling, and the like to the health sector. These taxes have produced revenues that expand with incomes and inflation but generally they have not produced large amounts of money. In several countries in the Americas and in Asia, lotteries have been organized to benefit social welfare programmes such as health care, slum upgrading, and primary education. Dedicated taxes should be evaluated on the basis not only of their contribution to the budget of primary health care, but also for their impact on the economy and their administrative costs.

Direct government financing of health activities alone has been inadequate in many countries. While in theory one might be able to develop a system of taxation that would provide sufficient

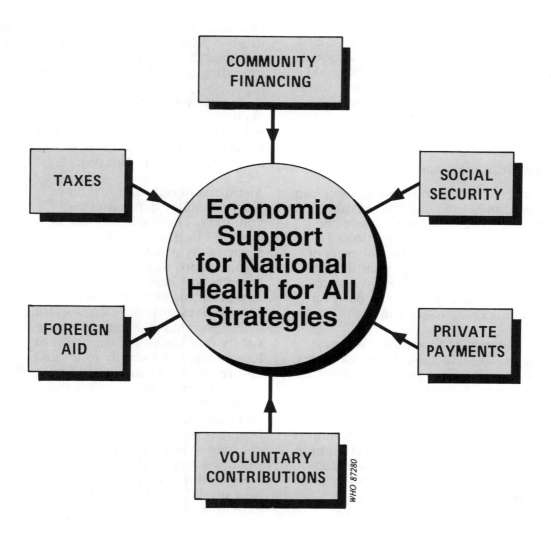

funds to meet public needs, few developing countries have the administrative apparatus to make such a system function. It has been estimated that as much as 70% of the economic activity of some South Asian countries is not recorded or recognized for tax purposes. In addition, as noted above, governments of less developed countries rely heavily on indirect taxes which adversely affect the poor who spend a large share of their income on taxable goods.

Health insurance

A variety of insurance mechanisms can be used to help finance the health services rendered to individuals and families. These entail collection of funds directly from potential users of the health care system, either to pay the providers for their services or to reimburse users in full or in part, for payments made to providers.

The advantage of insurance is that it converts unpredictable future expenses into payments that can be budgeted for in advance. A major objection to charging the sick for the services that they require is that the need for health services is a random event. The outlays required to treat even relatively simple diseases may often exceed the cash savings of most households. In order to reduce the financial crisis that accidents or illness might impose, households pool these risks. The agreements convert large, infrequent and unpredictable expenditures into smaller, periodic payments. These payments are collected to form a pool of resources that can be drawn upon to meet the needs of a participant who encounters misfortune.

Mechanisms to share risks and to facilitate the financing of routine services are needed regardless of the nature of the health care system. Where services are provided by public facilities, these needs are met implicitly by collection of taxes and disbursement of public funds to pay for the costs of providing care. On the other hand, privately operated health care, financed by fees from patients, requires an explicit programme to promote risk-sharing. This programme must attract persons with a range of risks and needs if it is to succeed.

Membership of health insurance schemes can be compulsory or voluntary. These schemes can be operated by government, by statutory agencies, by profit-making organizations (including company schemes for their own employees), or non-profit organizations, such as cooperatives or benevolent societies. These private organizations may be tightly regulated by government or loosely regulated simply to try and ensure actuarial soundness. The insuring agency may employ the providers of health care and own facilities, such as health centres and hospitals (the direct method), or contract with health care providers – public or private (the indirect method). Nearly all developed countries that now provide the same rights to health care to the whole population went through an evolutionary stage of voluntary followed by compulsory health insurance.

Compulsory health insurance or social security
These schemes are generally financed by employers' and/or employees'

Box 9   Main advantages of compulsory health insurance
of employees

■ The money is administratively easier to collect than an income tax.
■ The compulsory contribution varies with income and is thus preferable
in terms of equity to many of the indirect taxes used in developing
countries for a high proportion of revenue.
■ Contributions are more readily paid than taxes because the benefit to
the payer is easily visible.
■ The health insurance scheme can be used to negotiate favourable
terms for the provision of services from the private sector and require
cost-effective provisions such as a limited list of essential drugs.
■ If the insured can be made to pay for the full costs of the services
they and their dependants use, tax revenue has only to provide for the
uninsured. Thus the introduction of a compulsory health insurance
scheme can release tax money to develop and improve services for
those who are unserved or underserved.

contributions calculated as a percentage of pay roll. There may also be a subsidy from taxation. Compulsory insurance schemes may cover only the employees or their dependants (spouse and children) as well. Schemes may also extend to cover the self-employed on a compulsory or voluntary basis. However, it is extremely difficult, even in developed countries, to collect compulsory contributions from the self-employed.

The introduction of a system for collecting compulsory health insurance contributions is a major administrative operation. Several countries have covered first the larger employers, and then have gradually extended the scheme to smaller employers. Many developing countries are already collecting money from employers for provident funds or schemes covering industrial injuries. The additional administrative cost of expanding such a collection system to cover compulsory health insurance as well would be much less than where health insurance is the first or only social security scheme.

Countries' experience with compulsory insurance has revealed a number of common problems. In some countries, funds have been used to develop separate health systems, owned and operated by one or more social security funds for insured persons and their dependants – the direct provision of services. This can lead to wasteful duplication of hospitals, lack of equity, and problems of coordination as the social security system expands. Services run by social security funds can also, like government services, become inefficient, particularly if restrictive practices are developed by employee organizations.

Where service provision is contracted out (the indirect method), administrative efficiency depends on the terms of the contract and methods of paying providers or reimbursing users of services. A poorly devised and supervised system can lead to false claims by providers, incentives for excessive services, and a whole series of corrupt practices on the part of both providers and users.

Social security services, whether provided by the direct or the indirect method, can also generate financial incentives for scarce trained health manpower to leave government services and concentrate on providing curative services in urban areas. However, this can be avoided if terms of service are devised by or in close coordination with ministries of health. There are examples throughout the world of social security-finance schemes, using direct or indirect methods or some combination of the two, which provide comprehensive, good-quality care efficiently and at an acceptable cost.

Ministries of finance may be opposed to the introduction of compulsory health insurance on the grounds that it will raise prices, generate inflation and damage exports. It may be argued that employers are likely, at least in the short term, to add the cost of their contributions to the prices of the goods they produce and that employees may be induced by the payment of contributions to seek higher pay. These arguments however assume that employers are spending nothing on health care and that employees are not already buying health care in the private sector. To be offset against the cost of compulsory health insurance are the savings to employers from reducing their existing commitments for the health of their employees and the savings to employees from purchasing in the private sector. Surveys may well need to be made to quantify those savings and convince ministries of finance that the savings really will be made.

Some countries may not yet be in a position to undertake the complex task of establishing a formal compulsory health insurance scheme. Instead they may require by law certain designated large employers either to provide defined health services or to insure their employees in designated schemes of health insurance where they exist or can readily be established. Such legal requirements have been imposed for many years in some developing countries, particularly in the case of mines and agricultural estates. The law may specify that a stated proportion of the payroll must be spent on the health care of employees. Care is needed to see that these provisions do not conflict with national priorities, are not wasteful of scarce resources, are not socially divisive in local communities, and are coordinated with national developments.

Voluntary insurance

People may be allowed to be voluntary contributors to a social security scheme, run by government or statutory agencies, which is compulsory for others. Alternatively, they may insure with profit or non-profit agencies or they may join a group scheme.

Box 10 Singapore's family savings scheme

Faced with mounting costs of the medical services, the Ministry of Health of Singapore started to look at various options for changing the health financing system. The problem was to keep the balance between demand and supply capacity. With growing affluence and greater health consciousness, many people are wanting more and better services.

These considerations formed the basis for the National Health Plan formulated by the Ministry of Health in 1983. Its key proposal, the Medisave Scheme, attempts to impose compulsory savings and to restructure the system of health care financing.

In addition to promoting individual responsibility for maintaining good health, it aims to build up financial resources so as to provide the means to pay for medical care during illness.

Compulsory savings for medical care are regularly set aside by the transfer of 6% of earnings into a personal Medisave Account. Funds can be withdrawn from the Medisave Account to pay for hospital charges and some outpatient procedures, such as minor surgery, which are costly but do not require the patient to stay in hospital. Medisave does not cover general outpatient treatment, for which the cost in Singapore is considered affordable. Nor is it intended to cover long-term chronic illnesses, since other modes of care are already provided through subsidized government programmes and by voluntary bodies.

Medisave can be used to pay for the medical expenses of immediate family members. It covers spouses, parents and children, so there is a shared responsibiity in looking after the welfare of family members. It is hoped that Medisave will also act as a financial incentive for the entire family to remain fit and well together, and to avoid incurring medical expenses.

The Medisave Scheme was first implemented in all government hospitals in April 1984. In essence, Medisave serves as an additional source of personal financing for medical expenditure incurred by individual families. Wtih this shift in public cost-sharing, government tax revenue has been freed to meet other priorities and to improve the public health services, especially as regards preventive action and care of the chronically sick.

Source: Phua, K. H., Singapore's family savings scheme. World health, May 1986, pp. 11-12.

Groups may be formed by the employees of a firm or the members of a social organization, or may be determined by the insurer on the basis of age, occupation, sex, or other characteristics. An employer may insure all his employees. The characteristics of the group are used to predict the number of claims likely to be presented. Private insurers must recover the total cost of providing care, as well as the administrative costs, from participants. Thus insurance companies must guard against enrolling only those who are likely to need expensive health care. Insurance schemes typically require the patient to make an initial payment for care before applying for benefits (the "deductible"), and many also require the patient to pay a small share of the additional amount (the "co-payment"). These two devices are intended to discourage over-use of health care services.

Health insurance schemes can operate by reimbursing the consumer, or the insurer may contract and pay selected providers (the indirect method), or employ providers in facilities it owns (the direct method). Where the scheme operates simply by reimbursing the consumer for part of the cost of bills submitted by private providers, claims can become costly. Some insurance programmes have therefore set standard rates for common procedures, and have defined a limited number of "services" for which payment will be made. These moves are intended to control the claims against the insurance fund. The main criticism of health insurance schemes is that by distributing the risks and costs of care over large numbers of people, the schemes dilute the financial incentives to use health services sparingly and to resist high prices for services. A further criticism is that individuals with poor health records and thus major health care needs are unable to obtain insurance.

Schemes that offer comprehensive care for a fixed annual charge expect to profit by using preventive services and early detection and treatment to reduce the need for more costly institutional care. Thus they expect to be able to offer a wider range of health services at a lower cost. If a number of organizations compete among themselves for members, then the one that is most successful in minimizing the costs of providing acceptable care and thus can survive on the smallest fee, may be expected to flourish. Competitors with higher costs are expected to be driven from the market. Competition for customers can be expected to impose discipline and accountability on the provider organizations. However, for competition to continue to impose this discipline, it must be possible for new organizations to enter the market easily. Again there is the problem that persons with major health needs are likely to be denied admission into the programme.

In developing countries with little practical experience of the concept and structure of personal insurance, participants have tended to withdraw from a scheme if their benefits did not equal their payments over a fairly short period of time. This has left schemes with participants who have greater than average needs and has forced up the cost of premiums. This problem is

Box 11 Community financing in Senegal

Community financing in Senegal has persuaded people to take much more responsibility for their own health. To give just one example, the funds raised in 1983-84 by the system of self-management amounted to 80% of the budgetary appropriations, excluding staff, of Senegal's Ministry of Public Health.

At the national level, receipts during the first year of the project amounted to 303 million CFA francs or US$ 800 000. Community participation was responsible for the building of 115 maternity units and 49 health posts. In effect, the people and state of Senegal doubled their health care purchasing power.

It is the people themselves who manage this system, which is financed by patients' contributions. It covers all hospitals, health centres (department level), health posts (rural community level) and health huts (village level). The charge is 100 CFA francs per adult (US$ 0.26) or 50 CFA francs per child for treatment in hospitals and health centres, and 50 or 25 CFA francs for adults or children attending health posts.

These receipts are administered by health committees which include representatives of every health hut in the village, so they have to learn the intricacies of management; 60% of the receipts are used to buy drugs, 30% for staff expenses (female birth attendant, community health worker), and 10% for operational expenses.

The village came into its own again, so to speak, around the health hut. The council of elders, the rural council, the mothers' committees and the health committee all meet under the palaver tree to discuss their problems of health, hygiene, and cleanliness. They consider how to replace their stock of drugs and how to pay, in money or in kind, the community health worker whom they themselves have chosen.

Human resources have never been lacking whenever the need arose. Community participation finds expression in a thousand and one ways, including the building of health huts, and payment for care and essential drugs.

Some 90% of the villagers are making use of the health huts. Consequently less time, money and effort are wasted than before, when the villagers had to go to a distant health post.

Source: Sène, P. M., Community financing in Senegal. *World health*, May 1986, pp. 4-6.

likely to be greater if insurance is confined to major expenses such as a hospital stay of over a week. While such insurance may be relatively cheap, it is likely to be difficult to attract and keep policy-holders.

Community financing

The involvement of individuals and the community, in both developing and developed countries, has been increasingly seen as an important means of decentralizing decision-making in health matters, promoting life-styles conducive to health, and improving effectiveness of health care. A variety of mechanisms has been developed, often reinforcing traditional systems. Village development associations, welfare groups, cooperatives, and district health committees have been established to provide services that communities demand but cannot obtain from governments.

The emphasis of community support in most developing countries has been on providing resources, either financial or material and human, for the establishment or improvement of health and sanitation infrastructure, for example, health facilities, wells, latrines, drug cooperatives, feeding centres – or for payment for parts of health service operations. Some community health programmes – rural water supply, "clean-up campaigns", immunization, nutrition, diarrhoeal diseases, and malaria control – have been financed from funds contributed by the beneficiaries.

Spontaneous community efforts to develop or sustain health programmes indicate people's willingness and ability to pay for better services. People who invest substantial energy and resources in creating a local organization and then contribute the funds needed to sustain its activities have demonstrated their enthusiasm. Communities are likely to develop programmes spontaneously only if they recognize needs that are not covered by government programmes and have the necessary resources.

Where the government requires the payment of user fees for the services it provides, some communities have established funds into which village families make regular contributions. The fund then pays directly to the health services the cost of those user charges which would otherwise be levied on contributors to the fund. In Thailand, health cards are sold by village volunteers which give defined entitlements to exemption from user charges.

Sometimes community efforts have been motivated by discontent with the reliability or quality of services provided, such as availability of drugs, in local health centres. Community pharmacies staffed by volunteers have been established which collect funds from beneficiaries and maintain a stock of essential drugs. Alternatively, the government provides an initial stock which is kept replenished out of the revenue from sales (a "revolving drug fund"). These pharmacies are often operated on a commercial basis; drugs are priced slightly above cost in order to recover the cost of transport and of losses from pilferage.

Communities may obtain the resources needed to sustain programmes by a very wide range of methods. Many projects have imposed fees and charges for the services and commodities they provide. These fees may be paid at the time services are rendered, or may be collected in advance. Fees for simple health activities and for the services of traditional birth attendants may be collected in the form of produce – dairy products or chickens, for example. Cash payments are generally expected by modern health workers. Providers of care throughout the world accept additional compensation from patients for special services.

Informal insurance schemes have also been developed to collect subscriptions from people enrolled in a health programme or to impose taxes on production activities. The subscriptions are based either on the income of the member or more commonly on the number of family members enrolled. Production-based schemes levy charges roughly in proportion to the income of the beneficiary. Because the contribution is demanded at the time that people are receiving cash for their crops, collection is greatly simplified. Some marketing cooperatives, e.g., a coffee growers' group in Colombia and a milk cooperative in India, have withheld a share of each member's sales as a tax to support health programmes for members. Cooperative rice-polishing mills in Bangladesh and the Republic of Korea have imposed a surcharge on the processing fee, based on the volume of paddy submitted.

Community health projects also use inputs contributed by beneficiaries. These inputs include labour and local construction materials as well as cash. In-kind contributions have been used most frequently and successfully in constructing facilities. Some projects have employed volunteers to carry out routine activities, but most of these projects have encountered difficulties in sustaining the community's interest.

Community financing of health activities requires community organization. The most serious problems have arisen in trying to sustain contributions to pay for the recurrent costs of programmes and especially for the provision of sufficient logistic support. People have frequently been unwilling to continue to pay for programmes from which they were not benefiting at the time. Recovery of costs has been most successful where charges were clearly related to benefits received. For example, user charges for water supply and waste disposal are widely accepted.

Decentralization of responsibility and allocation of the necessary resources (especially logistics) is a prerequisite for successful sustained community involvement. While the trend is encouraging in many countries, resources remain largely centralized. With the current budgetary constraints, there appears to be an even greater tendency than before to decentralize decision-making on priorities and allocation of resources. Because of the critical importance of administrative decentralization, some countries have created new local or district administrative or legislative bodies, such as community councils or village community-reliance institutions with well-defined responsibilities and resources.

Conflict within community organizations can be minimized by keeping organizations small, restricting membership to people with similar interests, and pursuing narrowly defined objectives. Large organizations are more susceptible to conflict than small ones because the larger number of participants increases the diversity of interests and hence the likelihood of disagreement.

Governments can help local groups to organize workable community financing schemes. Assistance can be offered in setting up the organization and in establishing its system of records and its practices in handling money. Local organizations can be given authority to hold property, and audit systems can be provided to ensure that funds are used properly. In addition, women's clubs, organizations of shoolchildren, cooperatives and the like can be encouraged in order to give community members opportunities to develop skills in running local organizations.

User charges

Another way of financing health care is by charging patients. These charges are levied on those who use services, and take a variety of forms. Some form of user charges for health care is now applied in every country in Western Europe, through either compulsory health insurance or a national health service.

Water is often supplied through a public distribution system with metered private connections. The customer is then charged on the basis of the quantity consumed and a schedule of rates. These rates are often designed to permit families to obtain a sufficient quantity to meet basic health needs at nominal cost. Much higher rates are imposed for water used for nonessential purposes such as irrigating a garden or filling a swimming pool. In this way the charges for water supply vary with the importance of use and roughly in proportion to the ability of families to pay for the service. Water charges may also be levied on the basis of the number of taps or water-using devices in the household, or by the value of the property as determined for rates or property taxes. Property owners are frequently required to pay for the cost of pipelines and production facilities for water supplies as a part of the price of a building plot.

Fees for medical services are even more diverse. First, the definition of the item for which a charge is to be levied varies widely. A fee may be required for an encounter with the health care provider, an episode of illness or a fixed number of contacts with the health care system. A single encounter may be broken down into a number of items representing tests or procedures or goods supplied, such as drugs. The rates applied to each of these may also vary widely. A uniform price may be charged for all patients or for all except the poor, children, or other categories who are exempt, or a sliding scale of rates may be applied such that lower fees are paid by persons of lesser means. Prices may be adjusted by the provider of health care or may be based upon a certificate of low income from a local official.

The choice of chargeable items is crucial in determining how user charges affect the provision of health services. At one extreme, patients might be required to pay precisely the cost of services rendered. The cost of supplying a unit of the services of each health worker and each facility, and the cost of supplies and drugs might be multiplied by the number of units of each item that a patient has used. This makes the patient keen to ensure that only the services that are really needed are provided. It also makes the provider aware that his or her actions are generating costs for the patient. A set charge per visit would reward the health system for reducing the cost per visit, but would at the same time encourage further visits. Similarly, a system that charges for an episode of illness or broad activity, such as the management of a normal pregnancy, would shift additional responsibility on to the provider. If fees are based upon the procedures offered or the diagnosis, providers may benefit by giving more treatment than is necessary or reporting multiple diagnoses or complaints.

User charges have the advantage of providing a link between financial responsibility and the provision of services. This link has generally enhanced willingness to contribute to the cost of health programmes and has encouraged both consumers and providers to be cost-conscious. In addition, user charges help to control the use of health services by imposing financial disincentives on the consumer. Whether this reduction in health care utilization results in a better use of health resources requires careful evaluation.

The administration of user charges presents serious challenges. The majority of studies in developing countries have shown that the largest reduction in the use of services as a result of charges occurs among the poor. In this respect charges are in conflict with the aims of health for all and equity, unless effective safeguards can be developed to protect the poor by exemption. On the other hand, if charging for services enables money to be released for development of services for those not currently provided with them, then equity is increased. The major problems are to develop effective systems for exempting the poor and to limit the occurrence of bad debts that are hard to collect. Checking on people's incomes when they seek health care may be very difficult in societies where there is substantial illiteracy. People do not keep records of their income and much of it is in kind. Systems requiring certificates from local officials may work reasonably well in rural areas but are much harder to apply in an urban situation. Moreover, if health care services are needed urgently, there will be no time to be spent on bureaucratic procedures. In these cases, health care systems are obliged to provide care first and seek to recover any charges afterwards, leading to a costly process of trying to collect debts.

Nongovernmental organizations

Relatively unbound by the legislative and policy framework of governments, nongovernmental organizations (NGOs) have the flexibility to experiment with innovative and alternative approaches to solving health problems, often achieving cost-effective breakthroughs which could provide new models for national planning.

Box 12 Protecting the poor in Seoul

The Medical Assistance Scheme is a programme for the needy, 80%
supported by the central government and 20% by the local authorities,
except in Seoul where the cost is shared equally. The Ministry of Health
and Social Affairs sets the standards of eligibility for benefits, and the
local government is responsible for assessing cases and for day-to-day
management.

There are two categories of beneficiary, the indigent and the low-income
group. The indigent are those aged over 65, the disabled, children under
18 without parents or with parents over 60, and people residing at
welfare facilities; they receive yellow identity cards. The lower-income
group consists of those with an average income less than a certain
amount, and subsistence farmers. The level was set at 40 000 *won*
(about US$ 50) per person per month in 1985. People in this group are
provided with green identity cards. The selection of eligible persons is
made once a year.

The yellow-card holders receive medical care free of charge, while the
green-card holders have to pay 20% of the inpatient fees (except in
Seoul where they pay 50%). The Scheme enables them to receive
primary health care at private clinics designated by the Ministry of Health
and Social Affairs or from health centres and community health
practitioners, and they are referred to secondary and tertiary hospitals if
necessary. About half of the medical facilities nationwide are designated
for this purpose.

Though there have been occasional delays in payment owing to the
shortage of local government funds, the Scheme has been operating
smoothly to the benefit of 3.3 million people – 600 000 indigents and
2.7 million low-income people. This is 8% of the total population of the
Republic of Korea.

Source: Moon, O. R. Towards equity in health care. *World health*, May 1986, p. 20.

Nongovernmental organizations in
many countries have made significant
contributions to development of human
resources in health care and are often
able to mobilize critical financial and
material resources which can be crucial
to many developing countries. Often
dealing with specific health problems
or areas, they can offer concrete
technical support to government health
strategies. Some national NGOs have
been able to mobilize substantial
private, local and international
financial resources as well as human
resources (volunteers) which otherwise
would not be available for health

programmes. Family planning associations, organized women's groups, and associations for disabled people are some examples of the hidden potential for mobilizing resources in the community. Often a small government subsidy can allow the setting up of a voluntary movement which can more flexibly mobilize resources for specific deprived groups or a health problem that otherwise may not receive the attention it deserves.

While the overall contribution of NGOs in financial terms may be small in most cases, their potential for mobilizing people and strengthening their self-reliance should not be overlooked. In particular, they can support primary health care efforts by taking up innovative actions, especially at community level.

External cooperation

Of the approximately US$ 35 000 million available annually for external financing of general development, 8-10% is devoted to health financing. External financing is generated mostly through development-oriented institutions such as bilateral agencies, multilateral organizations and banks, and NGOs (for simplicity these are referred to as "donors"). Financial cooperation is generally channelled through a central authority in the recipient country, such as the ministry of finance or central planning organization, which coordinates foreign aid. In some cases, funds may be routed directly to particular ministries, agencies or NGOs. Conventions differ among countries on the extent to which external cooperation received from

government services is shown in government accounts.

Considering the large volume of external funds involved and the multiplicity of donor agencies, there is a need for coordination between donors and recipients to develop realistic and effective health sector strategies at the country level, and for both to abide by these strategies. Where donor efforts have not been well coordinated, recipient governments have been confronted by contradictory requirements and approaches by donors. Donors have, in some cases, disagreed among themselves on necessary sector reforms. However, there has been some movement towards consensus positions on issues such as: the importance of sector planning; cost recovery; institutional and human resource development; community participation and the role of women; sanitation; and health education.

Where donors sponsor similar projects in a recipient country, coordination of training efforts and strengthening of national capacities by collaborative institutional development are essential to secure better returns on investments. Countries with well formulated proposals rooted in a clear, national strategy, and with plans scrupulously in line with declared national priorities, are more likely to be successful in attracting external financing.

Because external financing is more readily available for capital investments than for recurrent costs, countries that have already received assistance for capital expenditures may later find themselves facing substantial recurrent cost obligations. This becomes a critical problem when current budgets are suddenly reduced as a result of economic stringency.

The mobilization of external resources requires a working knowledge and adaptation of the development financing procedures which have evolved over a period of more than 30 years. Donor agencies note that the health demand has by no means yet reached its peak. However, the health sector must organize itself effectively for the task of mobilizing external financial resources to realize the goals of health for all.

Conclusions

In so far as tax revenues for the health sector are likely to be tightly limited in all countries irrespective of their level of socioeconomic development, possible sources of financing include charges to certain categories of users or for particular services, compulsory health insurance (where it has not already been extensively developed), formal voluntary insurance and informal local insurance, revolving funds, and voluntary contributions in cash and kind. Local financing as a part of community involvement can effect change, and decentralization can strengthen managerial capacity at the local level. All these financing mechanisms to provide economic support to the national strategies for health for all should be considered and decisions taken on the basis of the criteria that have been suggested above. The search for further financing is, as shown in Chapter II, an integral part of the construction of a financial master plan.

What is clear is the overwhelming importance of examining every possible new source of internal financing and finding more cost-effective ways of using resources to achieve health for all goals.

Chapter IV

Making better use of resources

Background

Primary health care addresses the main health problems in the community and accords priority to the interventions that are most effective, scientifically sound, affordable, and responsive to the felt needs. Considerable energy has been devoted over the past decade to refining the health technologies that are applicable at the family and community level, either by people themselves or by health personnel with limited training. A health system based on primary health care should provide the essential elements of primary health care to the community. More complex health problems and specialized health services should be dealt with at intermediate and central levels. Organized in this fashion, health resources can be effectively and productively used. Furthermore, a primary health care strategy requires coordinated efforts with other relevant sectors, such as agriculture, education, and environmental health. Thus, adverse impacts on development programmes can be mitigated, and activities can be synergistic, thereby increasing overall cost-effectiveness.

Better use of resources is thus an implicit objective of primary health care. This is equally true for developing as well as developed countries. Health care systems in the latter have become complex and costly enterprises. The effectiveness of their impressive infrastructure and high-technology approach for meeting the emerging health problems of their people is debatable.

Cost-containment policies have begun to surface in many countries, reflected in health promotion strategies that emphasize and support individual self-reliance.

There is general concern in all countries that the available health resources could be used more effectively and efficiently. Comprehensive, scientifically sound studies of the cost-effectiveness of resource use in the health sector are needed. A large share of health resources (up to 50% in some countries) is wasted because of poor management practices, use of inappropriate technologies, excessive and unnecessary routine care norms or other factors and forces, not all of which are amenable to rapid change.

The issues are not only managerial but also ethical, political and attitudinal. However, the magnitude of the problem demands that urgent attention be devoted to this area in order to increase the impact of available resources.

This chapter describes some of the major causes of wastage of resources and suggests how better control of the resources devoted to health care can be established. Proposals are made for improving efficiency in the use of human resources, technology and disease control strategies. The third section is devoted to cost-containment, while the final section focuses on policy issues and responsibilities in this area.

Improving accountability

The major causes of waste of health resources are their misappropriation, underemployment, and deterioration.

Misappropriation

The magnitude of waste resulting from the diversion of health inputs is difficult to assess. However, managers know in general terms how important this waste is, especially in the case of drugs. In some countries, the loss of imported drugs can be as much as 70% from the time they are delivered to the country to the time they are supplied to the peripheral health posts for distribution. Inadequate transport systems cripple both the supervision and the distribution of drugs and supplies. Lack of regular provision of drugs and other supplies not only undermines the functions of services, but also discourages the use of peripheral health facilities, such as dispensaries and health posts. Relatively minor gaps in supplies can have a substantial negative effect on the productivity of the entire health care system.

The delivery of health services requires inputs that can be used for other purposes or readily sold in grey or black markets. For example, motor vehicles provided to the health sector may be diverted to personal use by health workers or unauthorized use in the transport of goods and passengers. While these alternative uses may be valuable to the community or individual they nevertheless diminish the transport available to the health sector. Stocks of spare parts, lubricants and fuels for motor vehicles may be stolen or sold for private gain. In remote rural areas where such goods are particularly scarce and administrative supervision is often weak, they are easily misappropriated. Drugs, bandages and dressings supplied by the government for free distribution or at nominal cost may be diverted, either by health workers or by patients, to private markets where they are sold to the public or used in licit or illicit private practice. Where unwarranted resale of goods works well, its major effect is to enrich those who divert and resell the goods. However, control over the prescription and quality of drugs typically deteriorates when unqualified and unregulated retailers assume responsibility for their distribution.

Underemployment

Despite the scarcity of health care in much of the world, many health workers and health facilities (including village health posts) are seriously underused. In many instances in rural areas, health facilities operate for only two or three hours a day, serving 20% or less of those needing care. Part of the explanation for underutilization of peripheral facilities is that too few people live within a reasonable distance to occupy fully the facility and its staff. Where transport is not available (or perhaps not affordable), rural health posts and dispensaries can serve only those who live within a reasonable walking distance. However, self-referral to higher level facilities (district hospitals typically) is also a major explanation for underuse of local health facilities. This by-passing of local facilities is often a consequence of the public's lack of confidence in the quality of services available locally. Other reasons include lack of supplies and equipment; harsh and uncaring attitudes of the health care providers; high costs or imposition of unofficial "surcharges" for services; decentralized decision-making; poor managerial capacity at the local level; and inadequate support and supervision services.

Deterioration of resources

Delays and/or bottlenecks from procurement to distribution may cause health workers to receive unusable medical supplies and equipment, including out-of-date drugs. If the operating budget is inadequate, health facilities may also suffer from insufficient maintenance and deficiencies in hygiene as well as substandard storage of materials. Local and intermediate levels of health care systems often lack the expertise required for proper maintenance and repair of equipment and vehicles, which eventually become unfit for use.

Formal accounting and management information systems can be implemented to enable supervisors to detect waste and misuse. Such systems are designed to record the quantities of goods made available and the activities undertaken by the health facility or health worker. These systems must be integrated in order to cross-check the accuracy and credibility of reports and allow rapid identification of anomalies for follow-up by managers. The development of inexpensive personal computers has made computerization of these tasks a practical option. Computerized accounting and cost-control have had a major impact on the management of hospitals, drug supplies, and district health programmes. Formal accounting and management information systems are also essential tools in the assignment of health manpower and the distribution of facilities and medical supplies.

Another means by which resource accountability can be improved is through the community. Community involvement in health services management can take various forms, from the simplest at the primary health care level to the most sophisticated (e.g., consumer unions; representation of local people in management committees). Close direct supervision of providers of care by the formal bureaucracy is difficult, irregular and costly. However, communities' representatives can successfully oversee some aspects of the operation of health facilities such as hours of service, use of vehicles, availability of drugs, management of funds collected or allocated, maintenance of facilities, and so on. For such management to succeed, the authority of the group responsible must be recognized by the community and respected by higher levels of the health administration. Prompt, effective follow-up of complaints from the community by higher authorities is essential.

The third point at which accountability can be improved is at the level of the health worker. On the basis of a clear definition of his or her professional responsibilities, the health worker has to be accountable to the community and to report to his or her supervisor for delegated responsibility. This managerial requirement is common for all types of service delivery and at any level in the hierarchy of the system. In primary health care, this requirement is particularly important as health staff, including village health agents, have to work in areas where close relations with their supervisors are limited and irregular. Thus, much of the responsibility for overseeing resource

Box 13   Kenya — a new drug management system for rural health facilities

Efforts to strengthen the drug distribution system in Kenya illustrate how improvements in organization, record-keeping, and management can improve the quality and reduce the cost of health care.

Only a few years ago, many rural health facilities (RHFs) in Kenya — health centres and dispensaries — were unable to give a proper service because of severe shortages of basic, life-saving drugs. Sick patients sometimes had to travel 100 km or even more to the bigger hospitals, suffering both physical and financial hardship.

In 1980, the Ministry of Health selected a list of essential drugs for the RHFs and tested a pilot drug-supply programme in two regions — one on the coast and one in the highlands. In 1985, the rural drug distribution programme functioned well all over Kenya, serving all rural inhabitants within a much shorter distance of their homes.

To save money, the quantities of drugs supplied must correspond as closely as possible to the needs of the RHFs. Standard drug rations have been worked out for a workload of 3000 new cases per year at a health centre and 2000 new cases per year at a dispensary. These quantities form the basis of the drug ration kits.

Ration kits

To avoid wastage and loss, the standard drug rations are packed at the factory into strong, sealed cardboard cartons which are not opened until they reach their final destination. The headquarters drug management team is responsible for dispatching the kits to the district hospitals in government-chartered lorries. The district health management team uses its own vehicles to transport the kits to the health centres and dispensaries in its area.

Health centres receive two kits containing a total of 38 drugs; dispensaries receive two kits containing a total of 31 drugs. The difference reflects the fact that clinical officers who are in charge of health centres have a more advanced training than community nurses, who are in charge of dispensaries. Since the system of kits was introduced, wastage and loss have been negligible.

Control

Drug supplies for the rural programme are subject to strict controls at all stages of their journey from supplier to user. The suppliers receive precise instructions as to the drugs to be supplied, their packaging,   (Cont.)

Box 13 (Cont.)

labelling and quality. Random sampling is also performed by the headquarters management unit, which regularly takes out one package of each item in a kit received at the Central Medical Stores, for independent analysis organized by UNICEF.

Outpatient register

Registers kept at every RHF record how the health worker is managing the patient. They include all the patient's particulars, the diagnosis, the treatment given and details of any possible referral. Part of the District Clinical Officer's responsibility is to check the register and discourage symptomatic treatment (treatment should be given only for a specific diagnosis and provide on-the-job training of health workers). Polypharmacy — giving more than one drug at a time — is also discouraged.

Benefits

The new drug management system has cut down the cost of suplying drugs to the entire population of Kenya to US$ 0.29 per person through such factors as bulk procurement in generic form, standardized treatment schedules that reduce the number of drugs prescribed, and the virtual elimination of wastage and loss. The service given at RHFs, of which there are over 900, has improved and the staff find greater satisfaction in their work.

Control of each individual drug on the essential drugs list for the RHFs has become possible for the first time. Finally, the supply to the RHFs is constant. Even the problems of the rainy season can be overcome by making extra deliveries in advance.

Adapted from: Kenya: rural drug distribution programme, *WHO Action Programme on Essential Drugs and Vaccines, 1985*

use and quality of services rests with the health worker. Efforts to recognize their performance, to instil pride in services and develop skills are likely to enhance professionalism and a sense of personal responsibility and accountability. The support services required to improve effectiveness in primary health care are described in greater depth later in this chapter.

The success of all these measures will depend on the extent of delegation of responsibilities in the health management system. Appropriate delegation of responsibilities requires decentralization in decision-making, adequate managerial capacity at the local level, and a strong support and supervision system. The crucial point here is to give sufficient authority to health managers to achieve accountability for responsibilities assigned to them.

Improving efficiency

The factors that affect efficient use of resources by the health sector are many and varied. Some of them are discussed in this section.

Cost-efficient access

If access to services were more equitable, the efficiency of health care would generally be greater. The importance of this issue varies widely. Where people have no access to services, the first challenge is progressively to provide to the majority of people at least the essential health services which have a low cost but are effective. When coverage has increased, efforts should focus on the underprivileged and the most vulnerable risk groups. Priority-setting for health programmes and the allocation of funds and resources should be based upon judgements of political viability, financial feasibility, technical efficacy, sociocultural acceptability, and administrative and managerial capacity.

Decisions about the location and the scale of new facilities are based generally on the costs to the responsible agency. The costs to households of travel, food and lodging required to obtain health services or drinking-water are usually not considered, though they may be very large in relation to incomes. If these costs are recognized in planning investments, higher levels of service are frequently found to be justified. For example, collection of water for domestic use in arid areas of Africa and south Asia takes several hours a day. Improved accessibility of supplies through an increased number and proximity of wells would substantially improve the welfare of households, even if they were required to pay the additional costs. Public standposts in urban areas are often too few in number and inconveniently located. Increasing the number of delivery points and reducing the distance from the standpost to the place where water will be used would in many instances substantially reduce the costs to households of meeting basic needs for water. Improvements would reduce both time and transport requirements.

The poor geographic distribution of health services also imposes heavy costs on consumers. Often patients and family members who accompany them must obtain transport to, and then stay at, a health facility. If, as is typical in rural areas of developing countries, transport facilities are limited and public services are infrequent, then the costs of seeking care may be very high for the family. The frequent by-passing of dispensaries and rural health centres and overuse of district and regional hospitals are largely due to the fact that the cost to patients is generally lower despite greater distances. The lower-level facilities frequently have to refer patients upwards because of lack of skills or of drugs and supplies. Careful analyses are needed to identify the optimal range of services to be provided locally, and rigorous efforts are required to ensure that local health facilities, such as dispensaries and health centres, are supplied and staffed adequately to be able to meet a high proportion of demands.

Efficient use of human resources

The issues underlying the various strategies for improving efficiency in the health manpower field are largely economic. That is, the cost of a particular type of health service may be excessive because the service is staffed by personnel who are more expensive than necessary or because its patterns of work are wasteful. In other words, the goal of efficiency in health manpower implies that the cost of providing a given service should be no higher than is necessary or reasonable for its proper performance. Hence, if a briefly trained and modestly salaried health worker can give an immunization satisfactorily, it is wasteful and inefficient to have an expensively trained and highly paid health professional do it. The use of a less expensive health worker may, however, require closer supervision and various other conditions for assuring that the work is properly done; the costs of these factors must be recognized.

Even in the most affluent developed countries, there have been many reasons for governments and community leaders to search for maximum efficiency in the training and use of health personnel. In many developing countries, insufficient human resources on the one hand and their inequitable distribution on the other can create a two-edged problem of inefficiency. In a growing number of countries in Latin America and Asia in particular, a large number of physicians in urban areas are either underemployed or unemployed. Considering the investment in their training, this is a serious wastage of resources which no country can afford.

In spite of these known deficiencies, most countries have not adopted adequate policies or measures to reduce waste in order to improve efficiency or performance. Many options are available for achieving greater efficiency in the use of human resources. These in fact form the fundamental principles of primary health care.

For example, one option is to promote the role of individuals and family in preventive and health promotion measures. This requires education and information support. In a number of developed countries increasing attention is being given to health promotion aimed at improving life-styles and health practices of individuals, thus reducing health risks and ultimately the demand for health care services.

A second option is to make rational use of health personnel consistent with the functions of each level of the health care system. For example, at the home and community levels, use of community health workers and traditional health practitioners, such as traditional midwives (wherever applicable), can be promoted. This option has to be carefully costed, taking into account costs of training, supervision, and remuneration.

Auxiliary health workers and middle-level health professionals (nurses, midwives, public health inspectors) have been used successfully at the local and intermediate levels of the health care system. Yet in many areas, these health workers are insufficient in number or inadequately prepared. Consequently, fully qualified doctors are carrying out activities that

Box 14 **The Egyptian dayas**

In Egypt, traditional birth attendants called dayas have for a long time demonstrated a great capacity for providing midwifery services among the population. In many rural places there are 0.4 - 0.7 dayas per 1000 population and some surveys have shown that they perform between 50 and 75 deliveries per year. They have a high status in the community and their advice is highly regarded.

Therefore, in order to reduce neonatal and maternal mortality through improved antenatal and postnatal care and safer delivery practice, the Government decided to develop an important programme to make better use of dayas. This programme started in 1982 on a trial basis in four districts and the process for extension is now proceeding very smoothly on the whole.

The objectives of this programme are:

a) to upgrade the knowledge and skills of the dayas in midwifery techniques as well as in other areas of maternal and child health (immunization, management of diarrhoeal diseases, family planning, maternal/child nutrition, community health education);

b) to foster stronger and closer working relationships with the health services personnel; and

c) to promote a broader role for the dayas as health agents in primary maternal care.

The following are some striking characteristics of this programme as observed in a recent assessment:

a) The health personnel at all levels have become extremely positive; the doctors both in the Rural Health Unit (RHU) and in the hospital are supportive and motivated. This is a definite sign of success of the programme.

b) The dayas have been eager to participate and acknowledged the need to correct bad practices. They have also given multiple examples of timely referrals for complications. They have been very willing and able to accept a wider voluntary role in health, particularly in relation to immunization, antenatal care and family planning.

c) The RHU supervision of dayas, the motivation of the programme staff and the perceived improvements seem to have been greatly rewarding. Receipt of a certificate and distribution of midwife kits were essential incentives.

(Cont.)

Box 14 (Cont.)

d) The process for developing the curriculum for the dayas' training has been a flexible and participatory one. The learning objectives have deliberately been kept somewhat general in order to allow this process.

e) The daya's training programme was not only making use of the daya and linking her with the health team, but was also a real strengthening of the supervision capacity and of the back-up capacity at the first referral level.

This last result is extremely important, since it is clear that, in the future, the number and the use of dayas will decrease with "modernization" and the demand for midwifery and obstetric services from the Rural Health Unit will increase. This training programme is really preparing a much more comprehensive move towards primary care with the strong support of the district medical team. However, the use of dayas is currently considered as the most cost-effective way to provide primary maternal care and also the most acceptable for the rural population.

Source: Edstrom, K. Assessment of the expansion phase in Beheira Government. UNICEF-supported Dayas Training Programme in Egypt, 1986.

an adequately trained lower-level health worker could perform.

No universal formula for the most cost-efficient mix of health manpower can be proposed. However, a health team approach, especially at the intermediate level of the health care system, can be advocated. A health team can help the personnel to carry out their duties in the least wasteful

and most efficient manner. The roles and functions of each member of the team should be clearly defined. The training as well as supervision requirements should also be considered. In this manner an adequate, appropriate, and cost-efficient mix of health manpower can evolve.

The potential gains from a more rational use of health manpower vary widely. In some countries the cost of outpatient care has been reduced by as much as a third by making maximum possible use of nurse practitioners, midwives, therapists, surgical assistants, and social assistants. Health post attendants, dispensers and family welfare workers offer the possibility of not only less costly care but much more rapid expansion of coverage, particularly in the lower-income developing countries.

Increasing the use of lesser-trained manpower requires action by governments. Training opportunities have to be provided, and in some instances, appropriate certification or licensing have to be introduced. Career opportunities also require expansion.

Pay scales may have to be revised and grades affixed to the new professions. Regulations and laws regarding the prescription of drugs and practice of medicine may have to be reviewed to ensure that the responsibilities given to the new categories of manpower do not violate the law.

Attitudinal changes are also required, both of the health professionals and the community, to achieve a more rational use of health manpower. Opportunities to train the new health workers in the presence of the full health team can help to modify old roles and assignment of responsibilities. Health administrators and doctors would have to acquire respect for the capabilities of other members of the health care team and support them fully in their roles and functions. Communities also need to be informed and educated about the roles and functions of the various members of the health team. Supervision and continuing education are also critical at each level to motivate field workers to provide a continuing service of high quality and to enhance their credibility.

Cost-efficient technologies

Expensive and labour-saving equipment which requires skilled maintenance workers and a highly controlled environment has often been purchased by countries (including developed countries) that cannot afford it. In much of the developing world the adoption of inappropriate technologies has sometimes resulted from aggressive marketing by manufacturers of equipment and from foreign economic assistance programmes that stress capital expenditures and tied

procurement. Sometimes, decision-makers have also actively sought highly sophisticated facilities in part because they received their training at prestigious international universities which prided themselves on having the most advanced facilities possible. Finally, in many instances the world market for simple low-technology equipment for the health sector has been too small to attract interest among manufacturers.

Excessive investment in hospital technology has attracted discussion throughout the world. Highly specialized facilities for preparing angiograms, computer-assisted tomography and the like are examples of facilities that are very expensive to acquire, operate and maintain, and that may not be used frequently enough to maintain the proficiency of operators. In the developing countries equipment has been purchased that is difficult to operate and maintain because of lack of trained technicians, inadequate electric power supplies, faulty installation, and high cost. Because of adverse operating conditions and inadequate maintenance, the equipment frequently does not function properly and deteriorates rapidly, thus requiring premature replacement.

The choice of technologies is usually made at high government levels. Indeed, the purchase of an individual item of equipment frequently requires approval at a high level because of the magnitude of the expenditure. Therefore, it is at this level that pragmatic decision-making is needed.

Decision-making about the choice of appropriate technologies should be part of the overall planning and management process. Ideally, the first step should be to identify priority objectives, feasible and affordable programmes, and then to define what is required in the way of staff and equipment in health facilities. Unfortunately, in many cases, decision-makers in both the developed and the developing countries have to cope with a heavy inheritance of large hospitals. It is not easy to restructure the hospital network and redirect the health system towards outpatient centres. Some developing countries have changed their investment policy by substituting health centres for planned new hospitals. In many developed countries, the results of hospital planning have been to concentrate high technology in a limited number of specialized hospitals and to devote new investment to ambulatory care centres. For instance, there is a trend towards redistribution of resources within geriatric care from institutional care to care of the elderly in their own homes. This is expected to reduce the total cost of the care of the elderly and to improve quality of life.

Within overall planning, the choice of technology should be made on the basis of the following criteria. First, the cost of an item of equipment needs to be assessed over its entire life in relation to its likely health impact. Then comparisons should be made with other technical options available, especially in the local market, for carrying out the same functions. Thirdly, the requirements for operation and maintenance should be examined to ensure that these requirements can be met in the future. If a technology is to be applied on a mass scale (e.g., jet injectors for mass immunization or handpumps for rural water supply), an evaluation of its performance under local field conditions should be made and design modifications considered where serious deficiencies are identified.

Because technical choices determine to a large extent subsequent requirements for operation and maintenance, they must be made with these implications clearly in mind if maximum performance is to be obtained. Similarly, because capital equipment often has a lengthy life expectancy, choices made earlier may have an impact for many years. Hence significant improvements may not be achievable until existing equipment needs replacement.

Cost-effective strategies

The efficiency of strategies (curative, preventive, educative, or promotional) might be improved either by reviewing the design of strategies or by strengthening support services for their implementation. Knowledge in health sciences and technology, and of concomitant cost-and-effect implications, has been improving steadily. Recent developments in diagnosis, treatment, and primary prevention have raised the need to reconsider the control strategies for several diseases.

Control of diarrhoeal disease and of schistosomiasis offers examples of what can be done. The development of oral rehydration therapy has revolutionized treatment of diarrhoeal disease. This safe, effective and inexpensive

Box 15 Cost-effective treatment of tuberculosis

The cost-effectiveness of alternative treatment strategies for tuberculosis has been studied in Botswana. The study compared the cost-effectiveness of a short-course tuberculosis treatment regimen using rifampicin or ethambutol with long-course regimens based on thioacetazone and isoniazid. Short-course regimens were more costly per case treated, but were half the cost per person *effectively* treated by isoniazid-based regimens because of higher patient compliance. In addition, outpatient treatment was much cheaper than a combination of inpatient and outpatient care. The study estimated that the cost of treating 80% of patients through an outpatient-based short-course regimen would have been one-third of that of the pre-1984 treatment pattern of combined inpatient and outpatient care and a long-course regimen. Furthermore, the number of people complying and covered by the programme would have doubled.

Source: Barnum, H.N. Cost savings from alternative treatment of tuberculosis, PHC Technical Note 86-11 World Bank, 1986.

treatment has sharply reduced not only the cost of rehydration but also the seriousness of the disease. Similarly, the development of an easily administered antischistosomal drug has made treatment of schistosomiasis an economically attractive alternative to the interruption of transmission through the frequent application of pesticides to the breeding areas of the intermediate vector, the snail.

A large number of studies have been made on the cost-effectiveness of existing and new diagnostic tests, drugs, treatment regimens, logistic supply (i.e., materials for ensuring the cold chain in immunization), mass screening, excreta disposal, water pumps, approaches to promoting healthy life-styles and so on. Appropriate practical research in the field of management as well as that of

technology is of great value for formulating and implementing national health programmes. What is required through this research is creative thinking to develop ways of solving problems.

The modification of control strategies sometimes requires little more than a policy decision. A major overhaul of the administration of the sector is not generally required, and problems of patient acceptance and compliance are seldom major. Ministries of health should continue to scrutinize the strategies being used to control specific diseases. These examinations should be especially rigorous when new technologies emerge, such as a vaccine or a safe drug. They should also be undertaken whenever the cost of supplying services changes significantly, more qualified manpower becomes

Box 16 An innovation in management development in Malaysia

Team problem-solving at the district level

In 1985, the Director-General of Health Services in Malaysia called upon his Institute of Public Health to develop a new style of management training which would raise the ability of staff at state and district level to diagnose and resolve their own problems, and thereby increase the efficiency and effectiveness of their services without requiring additional resources.

The Institute undertook action, using a learning-by-doing approach, involving, in the first instance, four state–district teams in the analysis, solution-design and, most importantly, the implementation of solutions to four assigned health service problems (immunization coverage, food poisoning, malaria case-finding, and management of high-risk pregnancies).

In February 1986, the teams were brought together for a ten-day workshop to facilitate their analysis of the assigned problem and to design and plan the implementation of their solution. This workshop included the analysis of existing data and some field survey activity to obtain more information needed. At the end of this workshop each team presented its proposal for action to a panel of directors who critically reviewed each. The teams were then given permission to implement their proposals.

After a period of eight months the teams attended a three-day evaluation workshop during which they reported to each other and to the same panel of directors the results of their efforts to resolve the assigned problem. The early results were impressive:

– All teams succeeded in remaining active and were able to implement their planned activities more or less as intended.

– One district was able, through special defaulter follow-up procedures, to increase third-dose DPT coverage by 50% and triple measles immunization coverage.

– A second district was able, through extensive health education and promotion of general practitioners and outpatient departments, to quadruple the notification of food poisoning cases. (Cont.)

Box 16 (Cont.)

— A third district increased the blood examination rate of fever cases in its malarious areas by 80% through the use of community workers, schools, and maternal and child health staff.

— Finally, the fourth district focused its attention on priority high-risk women and instituted an obstetric flying squad in its efforts to reduce maternal deaths, particularly those due to postpartum haemorrhage. At the time of the evaluation there had been no deaths from this cause in 19 cases, compared with seven deaths in 1985.

Impressive as these immediate results were, the programme directors were most interested in the ability of the districts to keep their teams active and working together, in addition to all the normal work to be done. Efforts are continuing by the Institute of Public Health to expand this type of management development and to assess the longer-term effects of such training in the first districts to be involved.

Source: Workshop for state and district health managers. Problem solving through the team approach. Evaluation workshop, 20–22 October 1986. Institute of Public Health, Kuala Lumpur (Malaysia).

available, or communications and transport improve significantly.

Strengthening of management support services

The strengthening of management support services (in-service training, supervision, drugs, logistics, transportation, organization) is crucial to sustain efficient delivery of health services. The provision of these support services has been difficult in many countries because the need for efficient managerial practices to deliver these services to numerous and scattered health units has not been adequately met. Support services are highly dependent on transportation and distribution of medical supplies and drugs. In many countries, serious efforts have been made to improve the management of essential drugs at each of the following stages: procurement, storage, distribution, supply, and utilization. Strengthening the managerial capacity of health administrators, managers and health providers is crucial to make programmes workable.

Another approach to increasing efficiency and effectiveness of primary health care programmes is through periodic in-depth evaluative reviews, focusing particularly on the managerial and operational aspects. Such reviews can take managers to every level of the health service and into the communities, in order to assess programme performance (including coverage, quality, and effectiveness), and to identify problems that may be hindering performance. Such programme reviews were initially widely employed by the Expanded

Box 17 A strategy to improve supply of drugs

Most developing countries import essential drugs, often from a few major multinational suppliers. WHO describes essential drugs as those that are most needed for the health of the majority of the population. There are about two hundred and fifty in the model list developed by WHO.

An essential drugs strategy can permit a significant increase in the quantity of drugs purchased within the existing health budget and thus improve the availability of drugs to the mass of the population. There are four important steps that can help lower costs:

— Selecting drugs and estimating needs. Based on the health problems in the country and the type of facilities available to treat patients, a basic list of necessary drugs and their quantities should be drawn up and kept up to date by the ministry of health. WHO's model list of essential drugs, which is revised and updated on a regular basis, can serve as a guide in this process. The ministry of finance, in its capacity as overseeing fiscal agency for all sectoral ministries, must ensure that the basic drug needs of the public sector are met, while at the same time being aware of the private sector's demands.

— Procurement. The lowest prices can usually be obtained by international competitive bidding, or by purchase through UNICEF. In both cases, foreign exchange must be made available on a regular basis to avoid expensive "emergency" local purchases of imported drugs.

— Distribution. Careful planning and purchase of drugs can help meet the basic needs of the population. However, unless careful thought is given to distribution, the drugs may not reach the rural areas where they are needed most. Packing the drugs in preset amounts in tamper-proof boxes that are then shipped direct from the central medical stores to the rural facilities is one way to prevent theft or misdirection.

— Use of drugs. Doctors and other prescribers must be made aware of the costs of their prescriptions, both to the community and to their patients. The use of standardized treatment schedules for the most common diseases is helpful, as is the publication of drug formularies and information sheets by governments.

Source: Catsambus, T. & Foster, S. Spending money sensibly: the case of essential drugs. *Finance and Development,* December 1986, pp. 30-32.

Programme on Immunization but were soon extended to include other elements of primary health care including maternal and child health/family planning, diarrhoeal disease control, essential drugs, environmental health, and essential care. This approach of joint programme reviews as a form of monitoring and evaluation has been found useful by many countries and has enabled them to improve managerial efficiency in the delivery of primary health care.

Improving cost-containment

Cost-containment has become a major issue in many developed countries which are confronted with ever-increasing costs of health care. Reasons for rising costs of care are many; for example, resources may be misdirected by systems of health care financing which provide incentives for excessive servicing. Insurance schemes that pay private suppliers of services on a fee-for-service basis are another major example. If the patient is not required to pay part of the bill, then neither party to the health care encounter has any financial interest in controlling costs. On the contrary, providers of care profit from charging higher fees and delivering more extensive procedures. Moreover, more drugs are frequently prescribed and more doctor-induced consultations are provided. Where insurance has been introduced without safeguards against these potential abuses, costs have risen rapidly. In addition, the use of more diagnostic procedures and increased hospital-based care have been common.

The rising cost of health care, without commensurate improvement in the health of those served, has led many developed countries to seek practical solutions to their fiscal crises. Recent figures show a marked decline in the growth of health expenditure in relation to gross national product. Many factors have contributed to this decline. They include a decrease in hospital building, a fall in hospital use, a relative decline in health professionals' income, more use of day surgery, a higher use of outpatient care and day hospitals for the elderly and the mentally ill, the control of pharmaceutical prices, the greater use of positive or negative drug lists, changes in the pricing of medical procedures, and an increase in the introduction of user charges. More and more countries have been placing budget limits on the growth either of total health expenditure or of hospital expenditure.

Influencing the supply side

One approach has been to revise the scale of fees paid by or reimbursable by the insurance scheme. Fee scales must be carefully designed to ensure that some procedures are not exceptionally remunerative and therefore encouraged. Very high hourly rates of compensation have been implied by fees paid for surgical procedures as compared with other forms of treatment and in some countries may have promoted excessive surgery. Relatively high rates for diagnostic procedures have also encouraged their use.

A second possibility is to shift the basis for payment from procedures to either encounters with the health care system

Box 18   Public health finance and planning in the Soviet Union

The Soviet Government takes full responsibility for protecting and improving the health of the population, under obligations set out in the programme of the Communist Party of the Soviet Union. The right of every citizen to health care is established in the Constitution of the USSR. The principles underlying health service provision thus include an emphasis on the preventive approach, the priority of making qualified medical assistance available without payment, the planned nature of health care, and the involvement of public opinion and organizations in measures connected with health.

The greatest proportion of financial resources allocated to health care comes from the State (made by the federal and Union Republic budgets), with lesser amounts coming from other sources including the collective farms, public enterprises, and other public bodies. The Union Republics contribute the major part of State expenditure on health, insofar as their principal concerns are with financing sociocultural measures and developing the local economy. In 1960 they provided 85% of all State health funds, and this proportion rose to nearly 95% by 1981.

There is a wide range of health spending among the Union Republics; in 1981 the Russian Soviet Federal Socialist Republic expended over 8 thousand million roubles on health, while the small republic of Estonia spent only 106 million roubles. In 1980 Azerbaijan spent 37.8 roubles per head on health, while Estonia spent 71.9 roubles per head; for Moscow this figure was 57.6 roubles per head.

State management bodies have pointed for some time to the need for more efficient use of resources in all branches of the national economy. This requirement has been addressed in several ways within the health sector. The principal measures involve the refinement of financial standards and the extension of the authority of the heads of medical establishments over the use of budget allocations.

In 1977 the national ministries of health and finance made joint proposals to State control bodies for changes in the financial standards, to make them consistent with developments in medical science and the medical industry, and in criteria for patient care. The Government accepted these proposals and increases were made in expenditure standards for catering and the purchase of drugs and dressings in nearly all health care institutions: maternity homes; provincial, territorial and republic children's hospitals; the clinics of research institutes; cancer   (Cont.)

Box 18 (Cont.)

hospitals; urban and district centre hospitals; heart, chest, surgical and other specialized institutions. A further increase in expenditure standards was made in 1983 for the purchase of equipment and drugs and for the feeding of patients in specialized care wards. Local health service management bodies and the corresponding subdivisions of the Ministry of Finance monitor the use of budgetary allocations by all establishments, to ensure conformity with the standards that have been set out.

Source: Golovoteev, V.V. & Pustovoj, I.V., Public health finance and planning in the Soviet Union, *World Health Statistics Quarterly*, Vol. 37, No. 4, 1984, pp. 364-374.

or an episode of illness or a hospital stay. This device pays providers for a collection of activities from which they may choose; thus the economic incentive is to expend as few resources as possible. The defect in this approach is that providers are rewarded for neglect and inadequate care.

Finally, direct regulation of the content of care has been used as a way of controlling excessive use of health resources. Review committees have been established by hospitals to examine patterns of diagnosis and treatment by individual practitioners and to evaluate the outcomes of care. These professional review procedures have not been fully successful largely because of the reluctance of peers to accuse colleagues of abuses or malpractice. Statistical analyses of patterns of resource use have also been undertaken by insurers in order to identify excessive use or possible fraud.

Influencing the demand side

One method for cost-containment and reducing unnecessary procedures has been to require patients to bear part of the cost of care. A nominal fee may be

charged for access to the health care system and a share of all subsequent costs may be charged directly to the patient. This sharing of the costs of care restores some responsibility to the patient to use resources judiciously and, at the same time, heightens the patient's interest in containing costs.

Providers of health services frequently claim that health facilities are overused by the "worried well" and those seeking to obtain exemption from work or other responsibilities. Patients also fail to complete courses of drug therapy, to return for evaluation of treatment, and to follow through on referral to other sources of care. The magnitude of losses due to such misuses of health resources is not known.

Misuse of health resources by consumers is in large part a consequence of insufficient knowledge of the proper use of health care facilities. Problems of non-compliance may also result from lack of knowledge. Health care providers must also shoulder some of the responsibility since they often do not adequately explain the rationale and expected

Box 19   Cost-containment in some industrialized countries

Cost-containment in health care is feasible and indeed, has already been achieved in some industrialized countries. It is a question of political will, acceptance by the public, cooperation of providers, and the use of effective methods. In a number of countries – Australia, Belgium, Canada, Finland, Norway and the United Kingdom – health expenditures, as a percentage of gross national product, have levelled off.

The following have been the most important cost-containment measures taken on demand or on supply. Measures operating on *demand* are described as cost-sharing – giving the term a wider use than is current in the United States. Cost-sharing means that the user has ultimately to pay or have paid on his behalf part of the cost, normally at time of use. This payment may be intended to discourage user demand or act indirectly on the doctor or dentist who authorizes the use of resources through the knowledge that the user will have to pay. The share the user pays may be a flat rate charge or a proportion of the cost or both. There may be a maximum charge and there may be exemptions. The charge may be related to income. It may represent that part of the cost which is not reimbursed to the patient – the *ticket modérateur* in France. The extreme case is where the scope of what is provided or covered by insurance is reduced. This throws the whole cost on the user (e.g., spas or pharmaceuticals which can be purchased without a prescription).

Systems of cost-containment operating *on supply* are of even wider variety and have in recent years taken more complex and ingenious forms when applied to contracted services. They include the following:

Short-term direct controls
Budget ceiling (e.g., for hospitals)
Controls on staff numbers (e.g., in hospitals or clinics)
Controls on levels of remuneration
Controls on prices (e.g., per bed/day or per pharmaceutical product)
Controls on quantities (e.g., the maximum number of items in a prescription).

Short-term indirect controls
Changing relative value scales (e.g., to make it less remunerative for a doctor to order diagnostic tests).
A positive list or negative list for pharmaceutical products or chemist substitution (to stop the prescribing of more expensive products where there are less expensive products considered to be equivalent).
Restrictions on sales promotion of pharmaceuticals to doctors.   (Cont.)

Box 19 (Cont.)

Information to doctors on relative prices of pharmaceuticals which are equivalent or near-equivalent.
Doctor profiles (e.g., indicating the number of visits per patient, the prescribing of drugs or the requesting of diagnostic tests per patient or per consultation) with or without sanctions for excessive use.

Medium-term direct controls and incentives
Controls over the construction or extension of hospitals.
Controls over the installation of heavy or expensive medical equipment.
Controls and incentives to develop substitutes for traditional hospital care.

Long-term direct controls on manpower
Controls over the number of students entering medical or dental education or passing into the second year of the course.
Controls over entry to specialist training.

Source: Abel-Smith, B. Cost containment in 12 European countries. *World Health Statistics Quarterly*, Vol. 37, No. 4, 1984, pp. 351-363.

benefits from a course of action. Better education in the use of health care and improved health education would reduce the misuse of resources by consumers.

Conclusions

Making better use of resources implies improved accountability, increased efficiency in the allocation and utilization of resources and effective means of cost-containment.

To reduce waste, underutilization, and misuse of resources, accountability must be improved. Information and education of the public are important measures to achieve better accountability.

Secondly, to increase the focus on the performance of individual health providers and of health care institutions, a relevant accounting and management system is required. Information systems have to be set up in such a way that responsibility for performance can be clearly established. Detailed, accurate information on costs should be made available to the providers and consumers of health services. Earlier chapters of this book have also suggested that programme budgeting and cost-accounting systems need to be introduced. This implies relevant training in accounting and management for health care managers and better organizational arrangements to review costs and performance in terms of effectiveness and quality.

Thirdly, to generate required changes in the delivery of services, lines of command need to be streamlined; and real authority is required in decision-making at each level of supervision and reporting. The potential for the delegation of responsibilities must depend upon the potential capacity of the various partners: individuals, communities, nongovernmental organizations, private institutions. Public oversight is needed especially for public health interventions such as vector control, epidemiological surveillance, and immunization. In order for consumers to oversee the performance of the sector more effectively, formal local organizations, such as health committees or boards, are needed in many instances.

In summary, the use of resources by the health sector can be improved by increasing the availability of information about performance and enhancing the responsibility and managerial capacity of individuals, communities, and health managers to evaluate and act upon this information.

Responsibilities and institutional relationships in economic support for health for all

Background

Health depends substantially on decisions made by individuals, families, groups, and organizations, all of whom contribute to its maintenance and improvement. Moreover, important roles in promoting and maintaining health are played by the health-related sectors such as environment, education, agriculture and housing. Participation in health for all is not just a question of democratic rights, it is an essential requirement for the effective and equitable planning and allocation of resources. Commitment precedes action, and the collective commitment of all concerned is required in order to ensure the equitable distribution of resources for health. Given the magnitude of the task of attaining health for all, and particularly of securing adequate economic support, concerted and coordinated action at all levels is indispensable. Action taken within any one component affects the action to be taken within the others. Hence, the shared responsibility which rests upon the individual, the community, the government, other national agencies and international agencies consists of specifying not what is possible, but what is necessary; not what can be done, but what must be done.

This chapter examines the responsibilities of different entities involved in health matters, the roles to be played by each in pursuing the goals of health for all, and the relationships between them. These include the government health agencies and other relevant agencies; the private sector; the community; the nongovernmental organizations; and the external agencies.

Commitment on the part of each entity is reviewed in the context of providing universal health care coverage, particularly where responsibility is shared. A coherent strategy for their participation in planning and carrying out programmes in primary health care and in managing the resources committed to the programmes is advocated so as to maximize economic support for national health for all strategies. Finally, the implications for the strengthening of institutional relationships and capability are identified.

Government responsibility

Much of the action required to meet the goals of health for all falls within the responsibility of the government. While no universal blueprint can be applied to all governments, the essential characteristics of health systems stated in the Global Strategy for Health for All define the means of developing infrastructures for optimum health delivery based on primary health care.

Governments' responsibility for health originates in the realization that individuals, voluntary organizations, and the private sector are unable to meet all health needs through their own efforts alone. Similarly, services that benefit the country as a whole should be provided without charge to individuals by the government. This would, for example, include mass immunization (the successful smallpox eradication campaign is an excellent case in point), and the control of vectorborne diseases.

National profiles of health and disease indicate the vast inequalities in health status that exist in many countries. The underprivileged form part of every country's population. People may be landless, members of minority ethnic groups, disadvantaged because they are old, sick, homeless, jobless, or inhabitants of remote marginal areas, or displaced persons. Most of the underprivileged in health terms are women and children whose well-being requires special attention within primary health care. The elderly are also vulnerable in many countries. Particularly in developing countries, these underprivileged elements of society are politically weak and are often too sick, uneducated, or geographically dispersed to become politically active. Thus, the responsibility for improving the prospects for these groups will fall upon the more privileged groups. Concern for the care, protection and promotion of the health of the vulnerable and underprivileged groups must be the task of governments, which have, after all, the responsibility for ensuring an equitable distribution of society's resources based on the principles of social justice.

The primary health care approach, focusing on the "eight essential elements", evolved in response to the mismatch between the distribution of health resources and health needs. Disadvantaged people not only suffer from poor health but receive poor health care. Conversely, wealthier people enjoy not only better health but better access to health-related facilities. Development strategies that are compatible with the primary health care approach contrast with single-purpose quests for economic growth regardless of the human consequences. Strategies that promote economic growth and reductions in social inequalities and increases in social services are consonant with the goal of health for all.

But government money alone will not guarantee the achievement of health for all. Political commitment and support are also critical to health for all. Indicators of the degree of political commitment are, of course, qualitative in nature and comprise the following: official declaration of high-level commitment; allocation of adequate resources (the most important indicator); the degree of equity in the distribution of financial resources; the degree of community involvement; and the establishment of appropriate organizational frameworks and managerial processes (including monitoring and evaluation) to move step by step towards health for all.

The importance of government intervention in the distribution and utilization of health resources varies with the service to be provided. The extent to which responsibility can be imputed to the government for delivering medical services versus the extent to which it should remain with the individual is continuously debated. At the heart of this debate between individual responsibility and social concern is the relative desirability of enhancing overall quality versus improving equality of access.

Improving the health status of the population cannot simply be achieved by governments expanding or developing the health services. Prevention and control of disease and the promotion of health must be part of a combined effort for the improvement of well-being as a whole. Thus, health care must be supported by improvements in the overall social and economic structure and contributions from sectors other than health. The health sector has the important role of coordinating these intersectoral efforts, by defining major problems, by suggesting preventive strategies, by proposing shifts in priorities and resource allocations, by encouraging positive action in other sectors, and by participating in advisory committees responsible for these efforts.

The main motivation for government involvement in primary health care has been to ensure that no one is denied care on the basis of income or wealth. However, this purpose is frequently not achieved, since lack of funds limits the level of medical service provided to significant proportions of society. Additionally, the increasing pressure of recurrent costs on public budgets is forcing governments to review the mechanisms used to finance health care.

Three areas of consideration are apparent. First, limitation of resources tends to diminish the quality of services provided. Next, financing through general tax revenues may cause a redistribution of economic resources from the unserved to those obtaining services. Third, those services that are available are not being distributed equitably.

One proposal for mobilizing additional resources is to impose charges on non-emergency users of hospitals who have not been referred by a lower-level health facility. In addition to generating revenues, such user charges would also discourage the bypassing of primary care facilities. In effect, the charge would represent the additional cost of managing a health problem at a hospital rather than at a dispensary or health centre.

Redistribution of consumption in the health care system could also be rationalized by introducing a compulsory health insurance system to pay for health services. Such insurance systems would levy insurance contributions on those with regular jobs who generally have access to services, but would exclude those who do not.

Individual and family responsibility

Primary health care originates with people and their health concerns. With this dominant role in health, people have to be actively involved rather than passively receiving care "from above". The rights and privileges of the people include the right to equal opportunity for health; the right to health care; the right to be informed; and the right to be involved. As partners in the health for all strategy people should have an opportunity to share responsibilities and to contribute actively at individual, family, group, and community levels. They should develop the ability to define and express their needs, with the awareness of when and how to use health care to satisfy those needs. They have the right to use the opportunities that exist to obtain the required information, to analyse it and to draw their own conclusions. Once people are aware of health problems they should have access to the knowledge and information that allow people to make choices in health care. The right of people to be actively involved in health care ensures that satisfactory prerequisites for health exist for all people; that their environment is healthy; and that their health care system is responsive to their needs.

People pursue good health and provide health care themselves through a wide range of activities. Self-care, for example, is the primary health resource in the health care system. Included are informal health activities and health-related decision-making by individuals, families, and neighbours, comprising self-medication, self-treatment, social support during illness, first aid, etc. Another term, "lay care", describes all health care given by lay people to one another in both natural and organized settings. In addition to family units, self-help groups are voluntary, small group structures for mutual assistance in satisfying a common need, overcoming

a common handicap or problem, and bringing about desired personal or social change. Groups may provide emotional support, information and advice, direct services, social activities, and pressure group activities. There is, of course, a continuing debate over the issue of self-help in both the political and professional fields, which could lead to a critical assessment of the quality and efficiency of the health care system in general.

In many developed countries national health for all strategies have identified individual and family responsibility as a key element. This arose out of the fact that health profiles of the population have changed considerably over the past three decades. Aging populations, health problems related to life-styles, changing cultural patterns, and burgeoning industrial development are a few of the factors conducive to rapid change in health profiles. Health promotion strategies under preparation in developed countries aim at enlarging the individual's responsibility in pursuing and maintaining improved health. Particular emphasis is placed on hypertension, cardiovascular diseases, tobacco-related diseases, etc., as conditions that are conducive to changes in life-style. Some countries, such as the USA, have achieved significant decreases in hypertension and tobacco-related morbidity and also in traffic accidents through developing and implementing strategies which emphasized individual responsibility and included active health promotion measures. The economic aspects of these modified strategies have not as yet been given sufficient attention. On the other hand, the benefits that have accrued already through individual

Box 20 Partnerships for health promotion – United States of America

In 1979 the first Surgeon General's Report on Health Promotion and Disease Prevention, *Healthy People,* was issued. The report chronicled a century of dramatic gains in the health of the American people, reviewed present preventable threats to health, and identified 15 priority areas in which, with appropriate actions, further gains could be expected over the decade. The report established broad national goals for the improvement of the health of Americans: specific and quantified objectives were established for the attainment of these broad goals and each of the 15 priority areas defined in the Surgeon General's Report.

These health promotion objectives for the nation are not primarily about disease treatment and control; they are about preventing disease and encouraging people to protect their health. The target areas fall into three groupings: personal preventive services, health protection, and health promotion.

Preventive services are those provided by physicians, hospitals, and other health care providers, and the targets are high blood pressure control, family planning, pregnancy and infant health, immunization, and control of sexually transmitted diseases.

Health protection includes efforts by governments, industry, and other organizations to reduce health hazards in the environment. Targets include the control of toxic agents, occupational safety and health, accident prevention and injury control, water fluoridation and dental health, and surveillance and control of infectious diseases.

Health promotion aims to educate the public about the risks involved in health abuses and increase public commitment to sensible life-styles that can add years to life. Targets include the health risks of smoking, alcohol and drug misuse, and stress and violent behaviour, along with the benefits derived from good nutrition and physical fitness.

The implementation strategy for these objectives and targets stresses a pluralistic process involving public and private participants from many sectors and backgrounds. Health officials and health providers must be joined by employers, labour unions, community leaders, schoolteachers, communications executives, architects and engineers, and many others

(Cont.)

Box 20 (Cont.)

in efforts to prevent disease and promote health. While the Federal Government must bear responsibility for leading, catalysing and providing strategic support for these activities, the effort must be collective and it must have local roots.

Source: Promoting health, preventing disease, objectives for the nation. Department of Health and Human Services, USA, 1980 (reprinted 1984).

responsibility in health make a strong case for economic support to such health promotion efforts.

Role of the private sector

The private sector constitutes an important component of the health system in many developed and developing countries. It is not limited to the provision of medical care, but is also involved in the manufacture and distribution of drugs and medical supplies, and in the provision of water supply, and sewage and solid waste disposal services. In the new approaches that are being designed to produce and finance primary health care, a broad spectrum of institutional arrangements to involve the private sector is possible. Different roles have been assigned to government agencies, parastatal organizations, and private firms. The suggestion that autonomous and profit-seeking institutions might play an important role in primary health care may seem surprising.

However, profit-seeking organizations already manufacture and sell drugs, build and equip health care facilities, water treatment plants, etc. Thus the issue is not whether private and public

health institutions ought to work together, since they already do; but, rather, how can governments shape relationships with private agencies in order to achieve social, and particularly, health for all goals promptly and more efficiently.

Private health professionals have an important role to play in all countries. Their expert knowledge and the influence they have in the health sector relative to politicians and the general public can be instrumental in mobilizing support and initiating change for the health for all movement. Further, they can accord higher priority to health promotion, disease prevention, care and rehabilitation than is often the case at present.

Of course there are some training, regulatory, and information roles that only the public sector can perform in overseeing and guiding the activities of private providers. The public health sector needs to take the lead in training health workers, testing them for competency, and licensing private facilities. The government must set standards and regulations to protect the people from unethical or untrained practitioners, especially where such supervision is not yet adequate through professional associations. Governments need to develop a legal framework for health insurance systems, and disseminate information to inform and educate the consumers.

Precise information is lacking in most developing countries about the extent of the private sector's involvement in health care. Even the term "private" is given different interpretations in different countries. Available data show that in many developing countries, the private sector finances over half of the health care services, especially in the urban areas. The role of the private sector and the methods for its full participation in national health for all strategies have not been defined in most developing countries.

At the same time, new modes of cooperation are also emerging both in the developed countries and in some of the developing countries. These are generally based on the financing mechanisms being applied in providing and extending health care. Some of these have been discussed in Chapter III. These experiences need to be carefully reviewed by countries in order to apply solutions that are appropriate to their own sociopolitical and economic situation, and that serve to expand the real economic base for the achievement of the goal of health for all.

Community responsibility

It is generally agreed that community participation is an essential principle of the primary health care approach, and no declaration on the subject by a national government or an international organization appears to overlook this requirement. However, development proposals generated by remote government officials often ignore these grass-roots systems. At the same time, there is widespread agreement that communities can play an important role in the identification of health problems and in the search for appropriate and cost-effective solutions. Where public funds are insufficient to extend basic health services to those without access, communities may be called upon to share the burden through contributions in labour, materials, or money. Community members have often been involved on a voluntary basis in defence of their own health. Some of the mechanisms being used by communities in financing health services have been discussed in Chapter III.

The political and administrative structure of some countries lends itself to local community involvement. Many countries, especially those with large rural populations, have long-standing traditions of community participation in all local development activities. The support of a variety of local mechanisms, often reinforcing traditional systems, has contributed to progress in local primary health care development. Conversely, low levels of education, differing customs or beliefs concerning the causes and nature of ill health, and long dependence on central government for all action and resources breed passivity and forestall successful community involvement. The emphasis of community support in most developing countries has been on providing resources, either financial or material, and human, for the establishment or improvement of health and sanitation infrastructures – health centres, latrines, drug cooperatives, feeding centres, or for the payment of community-based health workers. Important contributions have been made by communities in the form of volunteer services. Sustained community involvement, however, has remained difficult in most countries.

A clear division of responsibilities between the community and the health system, and effective mechanisms for mutual support and communication as well as administrative decentralization, are of critical importance in mobilizing full partnership for health promotion from the local communities.

Nongovernmental organizations

Many nongovernmental organizations (NGOs) have grown into national bodies, such as associations, clubs, and trade unions; and some have become transnational, principally through the rapid development of communications. They differ widely from each other and represent the most varied activities and interests. They are independent of governments and possess their own funds. Generally their aim, in the context of health care, is to assist people in the lower-income segments of the population of countries in which they operate to organize and utilize better their own resources, both human and material, with special emphasis on the local community level.

While it is difficult to arrive at accurate estimates of the financial

contributions by NGOs, health financing in 1982 by these agencies accounted for 18% of all health contributions and equalled the total input by the United Nations health-related specialized agencies.

Many NGOs deal with problems that are intersectoral in nature, growing out of such basic causes as poor education, poor health and nutrition, inadequate community infrastructure, high population growth rates, low productivity, insufficient income-earning opportunities, lack of effective community organization, and attitudes of overdependence and apathy that frustrate problem-solving competence at the local level. Since their motives are generally not suspect, NGOs can deal with these problems with effective, timely, and flexible inputs of relevant resources.

The growing awareness and wider acceptance of the role NGOs play in health care have resulted in a number of successful initiatives and projects which demonstrate the value of the partnership approach. Such initiatives include small-scale local voluntary organizations which may focus on socially deprived or underprivileged groups in a given geographical area, providing essential medical care, nutrition, and community education services and promoting self-reliance. Or they may be large-scale national-level organizations to whom the government has assigned almost full responsibility for a specific health programme. National family-planning associations provide excellent examples of such cooperation in several countries. Organizations for the care of the disabled also play a critical role in an aspect of health care that is generally very difficult for government health services to cope with in many developing countries.

The Technical Discussions on the Role of Nongovernmental Organizations in the Strategy for Health for All, held in 1985, suggested many practical measures for enhancing partnerships between governments and nongovernmental organizations. Nongovernmental organizations as operational partners can make a crucial contribution to the national health for all strategy and to international cooperation.

International cooperation

Many external agencies provide support to health programmes. These include bilateral agencies, multilateral agencies, including those of the United Nations system, lending agencies such as the World Bank, or international nongovernmental organizations and private foundations. In some of the developing countries, such support can be very significant.

Each agency works within its specific policy framework and operational procedures. These may not always be in concordance with each other and sometimes may even be in apparent conflict. When these efforts have not been well coordinated, recipient countries have been confronted by contradictory requirements and aproaches. Sometimes, the national priorities are influenced by the level of external inputs intended for a specific health problem or programme.

There is a need for effective coordination between external agencies and countries to develop realistic and effective national health strategies. Some countries have established coordinating mechanisms under one single agency, such as the planning agency, which serve to harmonize national health practice and external agency inputs and to coordinate international cooperation. Such mechanisms are needed in all countries.

Institutional relationships

Health care activities are supported and directed by both formal and informal organizations. In developing countries formal organizations usually comprise the ministry of health and its affiliated agencies, although organized professional groups may also have an important role in health care. Informal organizations are groups of people who organize themselves in order to establish health care priorities and to mobilize local resources. Frequently, the local organization for health care is one that was established for other reasons. These may be agricultural cooperatives, women's clubs, labour unions, or local units of a political party. Because marketing cooperatives are organized to promote local interests and have achieved acceptance, they have been successful. In some countries, administrative responsibility for local or district services does not rest with the ministry of health, but rather, with the ministry of local government or the territorial administration.

Box 21   Planning for equity in health – Zimbabwe

As part of the process for developing a health policy consistent with the economic policy embedded in "Growth with Equity", and thus based on achieving equity in health, the Government of Zimbabwe undertook a review of the health sector. The following is a summary of some of its findings on the overall structure of the health sector and some of the policy directions.

Overall structure of the health care sector

The Government of Zimbabwe inherited a fragmented health care system. Five subsectors predominated in the provision of "modern" health care: the Ministry of Health, local governments, missions, industrial medical services, and the private medical subsector. Various voluntary organizations were also making contributions to health care, most in specific problem areas. Each provider had its own character, structure and system of financing, and there had been little coordination among them. The most marked characteristics of the health care sector of Zimbabwe were the inequitable distribution of facilities geographically, and the discriminatory access to care on the basis of race and the ability to pay. The system had ensured excellent standards of care for a few, while seriously neglecting the mass of the people, especially in the rural areas. The style of practice stressed curative interventions by doctors, while the preventive and community aspects of health care had been weak, despite the broad scope for action to eliminate avoidable disease.

The primary health care approach

The Government adopted a policy to achieve equity in health. The policy emphasized the primary health care approach, broadening the social base of health activities and restructuring the health service from the base upwards. The policy also stressed the need for coherence between development and health policies and included as a priority for the government the strengthening of its institutional mechanisms for integrating development and health planning and for coordinating the work of the agencies responsible for health-related sectors, notably: health care, water supply and sanitation, local government and housing, rural development, agriculture, community development and women's affairs, and education.

Political decision-making and interministerial coordination for health

Given the close dependence of health promotion on socioeconomic conditions the Government has proposed institutional mechanisms for coordinating health with development policies action. It is recognized that the discussion and decision-making on broad policy lines on   (Cont.)

Box 21 (Cont.)

health-related issues take place at high government level. To provide a supporting technical mechanism to this level, the formation of a small intersectoral group of health and development planners is proposed. This planning group would call on the country's available expertise on health-related issues, drawing into a collaborative network the appropriate departments of other government agencies (e.g., finance, local government and housing, material resources and water development, women's affairs, and education), and resources of the university and popular organizations such as trade unions, women's and youth groups.

Source: Planning for equity in health. A sector review and policy statement, Government of the Republic of Zimbabwe, Ministry of Health, 1986.

A lack of information precludes a thorough analysis of the respective share of the responsibility and contribution of different entities involved in health matters. However, it is clear that in many developed and developing countries the public sector controls only a portion of the overall resources available for health programmes. What strategies, therefore, can be proposed for a coordinated and coherent approach to the provision of health care to the population that respects the principles of equity and primary health care?

No universal blueprint can be applicable for organizing institutional relationships of different subsystems or entities involved in health matters. This, no doubt, will vary with the sociopolitical organization and policies of the countries. What is clear is that more coherence should be achieved among the various subsystems and all subsystems should reflect primary health care as their major focus.

The successful pursuit of the strategy in countries will depend on one authority being responsible for directing and coordinating national health matters. In most countries, this will be the ministry of health. This does not necessarily imply direct administration of all health resources and facilities. It does imply the responsibility for channelling activities into the national strategy for health for all and coordinating them on behalf of the government, both within the health sector as well as within other sectors through the appropriate channels.

Experience is already emerging from several countries which have undertaken administrative and legislative reforms in order to pursue the integrated development of a health system based on primary health care. The short-term and long-term implications of these reforms and measures need to be examined in detail. But this goes beyond the scope of this chapter. It is sufficient to suggest that a careful review of the institutional responsibilities and mechanisms to bring about a coherent relationship among them would be an important ingredient of success in mobilizing economic support for the goal of health for all.

Strengthening national capability

In earlier chapters it has been suggested that countries need to strengthen their financial planning and management by establishing programme budgeting, introducing management by costed objectives, developing unit costs for a whole range of objectives, improving their capability in cost-effectiveness analysis, and estimating costs of their plans for health for all with identified sources of finance which are realistic and administratively feasible. This will require major extensions in the information needed for health planning and management, a development of capacity for processing and analysing financial and economic data and the acceptance by senior managers and planners of the importance of these new inputs to the process of decision-making.

Many ministries of health in developing countries lack the skills for this type of work, whether it is in

devising new costing systems, using macroeconomic data, applying systems of national accounts to the health sector, or making economic projections. Such skills may be concentrated in government departments concerned with economic affairs whose staff lack a knowledge of health concerns and who do not see the significance of health in socioeconomic development. Training in public health throughout the world, with few exceptions, has neglected the study of financial management and health economics, and particularly their application to the public sector. Where both economic planners and health planners tend to be particularly inadequately prepared is in the search for alternative sources of financing. Little may be known about ways of financing health services that have come to be widely used in other countries, and their effects.

Exchange and sharing of experiences and information are clearly needed among the national policy-makers and health administrators in this important aspect of their work. Training is also needed for administrative and technical staff who will work in this area. Skills are needed in the establishment and handling of financial statistics, in health economics, in national

Collaboration between various institutions and agencies that comprise the health sector is essential and should be based on clear allocation of responsibilities in order to make the most efficient use of resources. Countries should examine whether such coordination would be valuable, feasible, and acceptable and determine the most effective mechanisms for achieving it.

accounting and public finance, and in social security planning.

Research and development efforts on resource issues need to be intensified, particularly in developing countries. Such issues can be related to the allocation and use of health resources, the financing of health programmes, especially through new types of options, and cost-effective and economic analysis of health programmes. Results of such pragmatic research can then be applied to formulating or modifying policies related to economic support for health care.

Technical capability in these areas will require considerable strengthening in most developing countries. Research and health policy analysis will require close coordination in order to provide intelligent and sound information to the health policy-makers. Innovative approaches are needed to strengthen national capability in these aspects.

Conclusions

The strategy for health for all calls for organization and strengthening of health infrastructure based on primary health care, beginning with the individual and reaching to top government levels. Together with the mobilization, coordination, and rationalization of national and international resources, the commitment and involvement of people in shaping their future is a key factor. Where a mix of private and public agencies controls health care, close coordination and balanced decision-making must be assured.

Policy and institutional frameworks are needed in countries to provide a coherent strategy for full and active, as well as mutually reinforcing, participation of all potential partners in health care. National capability for dealing with economic aspects of health strategies will require considerable strengthening.

As countries reorient their health systems to primary health care, the need for change is evident. These changes go beyond physical design and may involve the redefinition of the objectives of the principal health institutions, the reallocation of responsibilities, and even the revision of the power structure. This presents important political and managerial challenges to the national leadership. Carefully yet courageously pursued, they would serve to expand the economic support for national strategies for health for all.

Chapter VI

Key issues discussed and recommendations

Economic issues influencing health development are varied and complex. They are closely linked to political, social, and economic structures, and environment of countries. No attempt has been made to cover the entire spectrum of issues. The following issues were selected to focus on what appears to be critical to the attainment of economic support for national strategies for health for all for a majority of countries based on the analysis offered in Chapters I-V. After clarifying some of these issues and exchanging experiences, participants in the Technical Discussions at the Fortieth World Health Assembly made relevant recommendations to be followed up and implemented at the national and international levels. These recommendations are specifically related to the four broad areas of issues discussed: economic policies for equity in health; financial planning; mobilization of resources; and making better use of resources. The recommendations in this chapter have been extracted from the report of the Technical Discussions.[1]

[1] Unpublished WHO document WHA 40/Technical Discussions/4.

Economic policies for equity in health

Background

Ten years ago, when the Member States of the World Health Organization unanimously adopted the goal of Health for All by the Year 2000, they endorsed the principle of *equity in health,* that is, shrinking the gap in the health status of the people and countries and ensuring equitable distribution of health resources. This called for a concerted political will and response.

The past eight years have been the most turbulent for the world economy in over half a century, seriously affecting domestic priorities and programmes in both the developed and developing countries. The adverse economic situation, which still prevails, challenges policy-makers seeking to achieve a balance between economic and social goals.

To protect the poor and vulnerable during the process of adjustment, policies and strategies of adjustment-with-equity are even more urgently required. The causes of disparities in health status can only be removed through intersectoral action involving the health-related sectors as well as resource allocation policies that give preference to the poor and vulnerable groups of populations.

Policy-makers in health need to be strong advocates for promoting social priorities in economic adjustment policies. They must mobilize commitment and support from other sectors and they must enhance their capability in defining equitable schemes of financing and of allocation of resources.

Issues discussed

The participants in this discussion group shared experiences in formulating and maintaining policies aimed at achieving equity in health. They discussed the process of arriving at such policy measures, including difficulties encountered and how they were overcome.

I. In the review of national experience, the following questions were addressed:

a) What has been the impact of the economic recession on public health policies in general: (i) in terms of priorities; and (ii) in terms of availability and allocation of resources?

b) Are there examples showing evidence of progress towards equity in health (in terms of coverage, target groups and provision of essential health services)?

c) How has economic support been given to make such progress:
    – by shifting resource allocation?
    – by changing the financing system?
    – by targeting resources at specific groups or health problems?
    – by other means?

II. Where the public sector controls only a portion of the overall resources available for health, what policies and strategies can be proposed for a coordinated and coherent approach to the provision of health care to the population, respecting the principles of equity and primary health care?

III. What specific actions would be required to improve the capacity of ministries of health in the analysis and evaluation of economic aspects of their national health policy objectives and in the formulation of policy options?

Recommendations

For governments

As part of cooperation in global development and in the spirit of international solidarity, the rich countries should make resources available to the poor countries on a planned basis, to help them improve the quality of life of the underserved sectors of the population.

In reaffirmation of the operative paragraphs of resolution WHA39.22 relating to the issue of equity in health, governments should:

- undertake an assessment to identify vulnerable groups, determine the risk factors contributing to the situation and respond through implementation of the interventions required from all the relevant sectors;
- undertake research on the socioeconomic determinants of health, the effects of improved health on economic development and the ,

effects of various economic strategies on health. Such research would contribute to the formulation of equity-oriented health policies.

Health policy should be negotiated and developed with the joint involvement of the ministries of finance and economy, planning, and other relevant sectors.

Adjustment policies based on empirically derived data should be developed so as to prevent negative effects of economic decline on the health of the population.

Governments should develop a policy for the preferential allocation of resources to those most in need.

Countries that have social security systems should be encouraged to earmark resources for public health programmes, in a spirit of social solidarity.

Programmes should be formulated, implemented and directed to the population groups most in need. These equity-oriented programmes should not be restricted to the health sector but should permeate all other relevant sectors through a combined intersectoral programme.

Countries should monitor the health status and well-being of population groups using indicators of quality of life.

For the World Health Organization

The World Health Organization should:

– intensify its support to countries to help them undertake the assessments required in developing the methodologies and indicators of basic needs. In this context, WHO should draw on the experiences of countries that have successfully developed such methodologies and implemented such approaches, and facilitate technical cooperation.

– extend the dialogue with other development and funding agencies to the issues of equity in health and the support required. WHO should also undertake an analysis of countries' progress towards health for all, and especially identify: a) those that have made and are continuing to make good progress; b) those that have reached a level of stagnation and seem unable to move forward; c) those whose positions have deteriorated.

– concentrate efforts on countries in groups b) and c), determine what support is required and, together with other agencies, try to provide maximum support to help them resolve their problems.

– promote intercountry dialogues involving ministries of health, finance, economy and planning.

– support countries in developing equity-oriented health policies and programmes aimed at those most in need.

– continue, together with other international and bilateral agencies, to support policies that they have promoted, and that have been collectively agreed upon by countries, thus allowing the countries to pursue the strategies to their successful implementation.

Financial planning

Background

Financial planning for health for all is an integral part of the managerial process for national health development. Policy formulation, programming, and implementation should occur interactively, supported by technical information, programme budgeting, and evaluative feedback. However, ministries of health are often poorly equipped to plan, allocate, budget and control their own resources. To a large extent these difficulties derive from government budgeting procedures which are more concerned with internal audit than with policy objectives, such as equity and efficiency. Certain other sectors share these problems, while some, such as water supply – which may be health-related – have better management information systems in which financial and economic data are important.

Where expenditure data are exclusively linked to budget-line items, it is difficult for health agencies to describe what they are doing in a clear way, consistent with stated policy objectives. Unit costs, even of major facilities, are often unknown, inhibiting analysis of the recurrent cost consequences of investment decisions. In turn, forward planning, the appraisal of sustainable capital projects, the identification of wastage or efficiency, and the monitoring of progress to greater equity, are all frustrated. A tradition of centralized responsibility for expenditure compounds these information weaknesses. National health development plans, which may outline a strategy for health for all, sometimes omit cost considerations, or build on unrealistic assumptions regarding resources.

To sustain a credible dialogue with ministries of finance and planning, and even more importantly to improve the value obtained from limited domestic resources for health, ministries of health should incorporate considerations of use of existing resources, and of likely resource availability in their planning.

Issues discussed

The participants in this discussion group shared experiences in financial planning for national health for all strategies. They discussed the process of developing such plans, the measures taken to close the resource gap, the difficulties encountered and how they were overcome.

The following issues were specifically addressed:

I.   Have countries been able to estimate the financial requirements for their national plans of action to achieve health for all? How have the requirements been estimated? What period do the plans generally correspond to (5 years? up to the year 2000?)?

II. If there is a gap between the requirements and resources likely to be available, what options have been considered and what measures have been applied for closing it? What have been the positive or negative consequences of these measures? Have these led to further readjustments of policies?

III. How have countries planned for the recurrent cost implications of their national plans of action to achieve health for all?

IV. What measures have been taken by countries to improve their financial management? What specific actions would be required to strengthen the national capacity in this area?

Recommendations

For governments
Governments should:

- develop the information required for the planning process by estimating expenditures and sources of finance for the whole health sector, both private and public, over recent years;
- estimate realistically the cost of their health for all plans reflecting their national priorities;
- explore periodically all possible new sources of finance for political acceptability and potential for savings from the more efficient use of existing resources;
- link their health plans with the plans of other sectors as part of intersectoral coordination;
- ensure that planned expenditure is in balance with potential income to allow for changing economic conditions;
- strengthen planning and management at the district level, involving all members of the health team and the public;

- publicize their plans to promote public understanding and to mobilize support;
- strengthen planning departments on a multidisciplinary basis with skills in health economics and financial planning;
- ensure that training in public health and health administration includes health economics, financial planning and management.

For the World Health Organization
The World Health Organization should:

- strengthen its capacity at all levels to support countries in financial planning, health economics, and management;
- stimulate the further development of training, procedural manuals, and guidelines in financial planning, health economics, and management;
- establish a mechanism for the exchange of information on country experiences in financial planning, and through meetings at country, regional, and global levels, explore the development of methods for financial planning and management.

For other international organizations
Other international organizations and national agencies of international cooperation are urged to:

- give greater priority to support for economic analysis and studies of health financing;
- give greater support to training in health economics and financial planning.

Mobilization of resources

Background

In a period of declining health budgets, meeting the cost of health services is for many countries becoming increasingly difficult. This applies both to extending primary health care coverage to all segments of a population, and to sustaining the existing infrastructure of the health services. This situation has led many countries to explore ways of mobilizing additional resources to ensure a financing base for the capital and recurrent public health budget and to permit more effective use of the services and resources in the family, community and private sector.

In the mobilization of domestic resources many financing mechanisms have been tried such as: government financing directly from public revenue, or through compulsory health insurance schemes (social security); private health insurance programmes, including those related to employment, cooperatives and benevolent societies; prepaid medical coverage, health maintenance organizations; direct user charges for services; community participation in cash and in kind.

The introduction of new ways of mobilizing resources will have effects – some positive and some negative – on the range of services that can be provided, and on their availability, quality and cost. Moving into this area will therefore call for careful examination of financing policies and strategies, as well as an assessment of the impact of the financing mechanisms themselves on health status and on utilization patterns, especially among the poor.

Issues discussed

The participants in this discussion group reviewed the lessons learnt from the experience of countries in mobilizing new resources by applying different financing mechanisms. They studied the measures taken by countries to correct or avert the ill effects of certain financing schemes. They also discussed the applicable experience of nongovernmental organizations in financing and revenue generation.

The following issues were specifically addressed:

I. The positive impact and the weaknesses or defects of each financing system with regard to:

    a) equity in availability and accessibility of care; social costs;
    b) impact on providers and the quality of care;
    c) efficiency and effectiveness of service, reliability;
    d) adequacy of available financing mechanisms.

II. The financing methods that have been preferred, by type of service, e.g., disease prevention and treatment, water supply, sanitation, maternal and child health care, family planning, referral and secondary medical care?

III. The organizational, administrative and institutional arrangements that have been required along with changes in financing mechanisms? What problems have been encountered, and what has been required to correct them? Where are the hidden costs in each financing method? Do the financing mechanisms actually increase the resources available?

IV. What has been the impact of external financing on the national capacity for mobilizing domestic resources? When external resources have been used for capital investment, what have been the recurrent cost and debt service implications, the consequences in terms of sustainability, the demands for mobilizing new domestic resources, and for maintaining programmes after the phasing out of external support?

Recommendations

For governments

In order to explore all possible means of closing any gaps between available and required resources for the implementation of national health for all strategies, governments should:

– establish appropriate mechanisms to achieve the maximum involvement and necessary coordination of all potential partners in health, including health-related sectors, social security agencies, nongovernmental organizations, the private sector, and the community, in order to ensure their collaboration in financing health development;
– evaluate existing revenue-raising measures and explore and try new financing mechanisms consistent with national health for all strategies and goals;

– strengthen the capacity of local bodies to mobilize, channel and allocate resources, and ensure that money raised by health services remains at the disposal of the health sector;
– keep under review the criteria and structures for setting fees and prices applied to the health services to ensure their optimal use and their equitable application;
– strengthen national capacities in financial management through training at all levels and by improved management information systems;
– establish clearly the requirements for local and foreign funds to implement the national health plan.

For the World Health Organization

The World Health Organization should:

– work closely with international financial and development agencies to ensure that a substantial portion of the resources available are reserved for support of national health for all strategies;
– continue to ensure that adequate resources for health are channelled to the most seriously affected countries;
– actively study, with other international agencies, and with both industrialized and developing countries, new options and possibilities for mobilizing resources for health, and promote the exchange of information and experiences among countries on approaches and options being used for expanding domestic economic support for health for all.

Making better use of resources

Background

In addition to issues concerning the economic implications of various health policies and strategic options, and the problems of resource mobilization, allocation, planning, and budgeting, the management of existing resources and services can be improved with benefit in terms of social relevance, equity, efficiency, and effectiveness. In particular, improved management of existing resources will lead to higher efficiency (greater coverage with critical services) and high quality, both of which will result in greater health improvement for a given level of public and private investment.

Issues discussed

The discussion on the management of health resources focused on the issues of efficiency, cost-effectiveness, resources accountability, and cost-containment.

The following were among the points discussed:

I. All health service administrators have at one time or another expressed concern that more services and health benefit could be derived from existing resources if only they could be organized and managed better.

    a) How have the areas of the service with least efficiency been identified?

    b) What steps can be taken to raise efficiency? Is there a conflict between efforts to improve efficiency and the desire to increase equity in the accessibility of services? How have problems of coordination, over-specialization, and integration of services been tackled?

II. Ensuring that the services and technologies that are given high priority during planning and resource allocation actually receive priority attention in the delivery of services is a continuing responsibility of management.

    a) What methods have been used for choosing the most cost-effective and appropriate technologies and strategies for use within health services?

    b) How have programme managers been able to ensure that their service providers continue to emphasize priority services?

    c) How have the most cost-effective mixes and uses of health manpower been arrived at and implemented?

    d) How has the *quality* of government health services been monitored, and what means have been employed for improving quality?

III. Contemporary health administrations in most countries are forced to deal with increasing responsibility in the face of escalating inflation and more stringent government budgetary practices. A waste of existing resources is an overriding problem which all responsible administrators are seeking to reduce.

a) Are there examples in which governments have successfully identified causes of waste in resource use and implemented corrective actions?

b) Are there particular cost-containment strategies that can be recommended?

c) What has been the effect of decentralizing managerial and financial autonomy to peripheral levels of the health services? Does the authority to utilize the fees collected improve efficiency and cost-control at these levels? What examples are there of community control over health resources?

Recommendations

For governments

Governments should:

– accord high priority to the orientation of their national health systems towards primary health care as a means of increasing the effectiveness of the utilization of resources. Active involvement of nongovernmental and private institutions and health staff should comprise an important part of this process;

– take action to establish or strengthen district health systems by introducing managerial mechanisms to provide for sustained coordination of all resources;

– develop policies and mechanisms to coordinate, where appropriate, total resource use (i.e., public, private, nongovernmental, community, etc.), so as to optimize the use of resources in furtherance of primary health care;

– define clearly their responsibility for improving the performance of public services and for examining impediments to this. The improvement in performance needs to be regularly evaluated with attention to the trend in service cost-effectiveness. Such evaluation should be multisectoral in nature. Further, governments should consider a variety of payment mechanisms at different service levels as one important way to increase accountability, responsibility and performance of public services;

– with the support of international agencies, develop or adjust indices that best measure the efficiency, quality and cost-effectiveness of different service levels, and this information should be widely disseminated and shared with decision-makers at all levels of the system;

– pay special attention in health manpower development to increasing general appreciation of the need for efficiency and cost-control, and to strengthening managerial and financial administration capabilities;

– employ new and innovative teaching/learning approaches, for example case studies on problem-solving, particularly at

community level. Economists and health professionals should jointly engage in such learning experiences;
- give careful consideration to regulatory measures that will be effective in controlling cost increases and maintaining an acceptable level of quality in the health services, public and private;
- use practical, short-term health systems research to generate information about health care resources, costs, service output and quality of care for immediate use in planning and problem-solving. Health service staff at all levels should be involved in such research, which should analyse "success stories" as well as difficulties;
- undertake programmes for better management of services for procurement, use and maintenance of supplies and equipment, through:
  - establishing procurement procedures, guidelines, and equipment standards;
  - strengthening maintenance systems, including maintenance facilities, and training centres for technicians;
  - developing training courses and materials for service staff in the proper utilization and preventive maintenance of equipment;
  - facilitating local production of spare parts wherever possible for widely used equipment; and
  - establishing standard drug lists.

Special efforts should be made to inform people about the personal savings that can be achieved through preventive measures and the best use of health services and technologies, including least costly medicines and service interventions.

Health education should also be focused on building public appreciation and trust for primary health care services, including those available in the community, such as home and day-care facilities.

When such health education is organized, special attention should be focused on the important role of women, particularly mothers, as providers of health care in the family.

For the World Health Organization and other international agencies

The international community of agencies should assist governments in sharing the results of such action-research, with WHO serving as one source of coordination in this exchange of information. The information should also describe practical research methodology and lead to the development of generally acceptable indices of efficiency, quality, and levels of health service performance.

WHO should facilitate further work on improving the use of health resources by convening special study groups and scientific working groups on these subjects. Of particular importance, and therefore recommended for early implementation, is the need to strengthen health personnel administration. A study/development effort should be launched addressing problems of health staff recruitment, assignment, career development, wage and salary administration, benefits, incentives, performance assessment, and discipline.

Glossary of terms

Accounting

The recording of income and expenditure, and of the balance between them, over a period of time.

Benefits

Gains, whether material or not, accruing to an individual or a community.

Budget

A plan in financial terms for the carrying out of a programme of activities during a specified period of time.

Capital costs

Expenditure on physical assets, such as land or buildings, that provide benefits over a period of years.

Capitation

A tax or fee levied per head of a given population, or a grant per head of a given population entitled to a certain benefit.

Cost-benefit analysis

A form of economic analysis in which all the costs and benefits of an activity are expressed in common monetary terms. This analysis aims to assess the ratio of benefits to costs against those of other alternatives or against established criteria.

Cost containment

Measures taken to reduce the rate of growth of expenditure.

Cost-effectiveness analysis

A form of economic evaluation which seeks to determine the costs and the effectiveness of an activity, or to compare alternative activities, in order to determine the relative degree to which they will achieve the desired objectives. The preferred action or alternative is that which requires the least cost to produce a given level of effectiveness or provides the greatest effectiveness for a given level of cost. The costs are expressed in monetary terms but some of the consequences may be expressed in physical units (e.g. years of life gained or cases of disease detected).

Deductible

A fixed sum, specified in an insurance policy, that is deducted from any claim made under that policy (and that is therefore paid by the beneficiary of the policy), the remainder of the claim, or a portion thereof, being paid by the insurer.

Demand

The type and quantity of service or commodity that consumers wish and have the means to buy in a given period of time.

Economic evaluation

A process whereby the costs of programmes, alternatives or options are compared with their consequences in terms of improved health or savings in resources.

Effectiveness

The extent to which an activity achieves its objectives (e.g., the adequacy of delivery of a treatment to the members of a population that could benefit from it).

Efficiency

A measure of how well inputs are converted into outputs, i.e., how well resources are used to produce the desired result.

Fee-for-service

A payment per item of service.

Fixed costs

Production costs that are unaffected by variations in the volume of output.

Goods

Tangible commodities such as vehicles, clothes and food.

Gross national product

The value of goods and services produced within a nation plus net income from abroad during a specified period of time.

Incremental cost

The additional cost of one programme, alternative, or option, over and above another.

Inputs

Goods, services, personnel, and other resources provided for an activity with the expectation of producing outputs and achieving the activity's objectives.

Investments

Strictly, in economics, expenditure on real capital goods (e.g., equipment, buildings, or roads); in everyday use, the term applies also to expenditure on other assets from which a return is expected (e.g., stocks and shares).

Marginal cost

The additional cost of producing each successive increment of output.

Monitoring

Continuous oversight (in the sense of supervision) of the implementation of an activity, with the objective of ensuring that input deliveries, work schedules, and other required actions are proceeding, and that targeted outputs are being achieved, according to plan.

National income

A measure of the monetary value of the goods and services becoming available to a nation from economic activity during a prescribed period.

Nominal fee

A fee considerably below the fee normally charged on the open market (by analogy, "nominal value" is the value given to shares in companies when they are created).

Output

The product(s) that an activity is expected to produce from its inputs in order to achieve its objectives; the quantity of goods or services produced in a given time period.

Prepayment

Payment made in advance giving a guarantee of eligibility to receive a service when needed at reduced or zero additional cost at time of use (e.g., insurance premiums, membership dues, crop share contributions).

Programme budgeting

Making a budget for a programme.

Real terms

Taking account of, or adjusting for, the changing value of money.

Recurrent costs (or operating costs)

Expenditure that recurs and that is not devoted to the acquisition of capital assets, i.e., the costs of running an activity, such as salary and raw material costs.

Revenue planning

Plotting future income.

Social cost

Costs to society, and not merely to the individual or agency carrying out the activity, that do not appear in financial accounts (e.g., the costs of air pollution, noise, congestion).

Subsidy

A grant of money to an organization or an individual from a government or other agency.

Unit cost

Cost per unit of production.

User charges

A payment made by the user of a service; it may or may not be related to cost.

Evaluation of the Global Strategy for Health for All by the Year 2000

Global indicators on resource allocation

Two global economic indicators on resource allocation have been selected for the monitoring and evaluation of the Global Strategy for Health for All: the proportion of gross national product (GNP) spent on health, and the proportion of national health expenditure devoted to primary health care. In the first evaluation of the Strategy, the use of these indicators raised some problems relating to definition, and availability and interpretation of data. Thus, the information that has been collected is not as valuable as expected, and in any event, changes in resource allocation in quantitative terms cannot be measured at this stage. There is still a need to develop additional and more sensitive and appropriate indicators for monitoring and evaluating resource allocation and utilization.

Table A1 shows the number of countries reported to spend less or more than 5% of the GNP on health. The number of countries that appear to have achieved the 5% target is certainly an overestimate. Indeed, some countries have given ministry of health expenditures as a proportion of the national budget rather than public and private health expenditures as a proportion of the GNP.

The data provided for the second global economic indicator are summarized in Table A2. This shows the number of countries in which a percentage of the national health expenditure is devoted to primary health care. However, because of the great variations in the interpretation of "local health services", it is difficult to draw valid conclusions from the table.

Table A1. Proportion of GNP spent on health, by WHO Region

Percentage of GNP spent on health	Number of countries and territories						
	Africa	Americas	South-East Asia	Europe	Eastern Mediterranean	Western Pacific	TOTAL
Less than 5%	21	13	9	9	15	5	72
More than 5%	3	14	1	26	5	7	56
Subtotal	24	27	10	35	20	12	128
No information	20	7	1	—	2	8	38
Total	44	34	11	35	22	20	166

Table A2. Proportion of national health expenditure devoted to primary health care, by WHO Region

Percentage	Number of countries and territories						
	Africa	Americas	South-East Asia	Europe	Eastern Mediterranean	Western Pacific	TOTAL
Less than 20%	4	6	—	3	2	4	19
20.0%–29.9%	4	—	1	5	4	3	17
30.0%–39.9%	3	—	3	2	3	1	12
40.0%–49.9%	5	—	1	3	3	1	13
50.0%–59.9%	3	1	1	1	1	5	12
60.0%–69.9%	2	—	2	—	1	—	5
70.0%–79.9%	—	—	—	—	—	—	
80% and more	—	1	1	1	1	—	4
Subtotal	21	8	9	15	15	14	82
No information	23	26	2	20	7	6	84
Total	44	34	11	35	22	20	166

Source: WHO. Evaluation of the strategy for health for all by the year 2000. Seventh report on the world health situation. Volume I: Global review. Geneva, WHO, 1987, p. 57.

Annex 3

Bibliography

This publication has drawn on a wide variety of sources. Major relevant publications and documents are listed below by chapter.

Introduction

1. **WHO/UNICEF.** *Primary Health Care. Report of the International Conference on Primary Health Care, Alma-Ata, USSR, 6-12 September, 1978.* Geneva, World Health Organization, 1978 ("Health for All" Series, No. 1).

2. **WHO.** *Intersectoral action for health. The role of intersectoral cooperation in national strategies for health for all.* Geneva, World Health Organization, 1986.

Chapter I

1. **ELBAZ, S.** *Economic and financial constraints and impact on health provision in Egypt.* Draft paper for the Technical Discussions at the Fortieth World Health Assembly, 1987.

2. **GOLDSBOROUGH, D. & ZAIDI, I.M.** How performance in industrial economies affects developing countries. *Finance and development,* **23** (4): (1986).

3. **GUNATILLEKE, G.,** ed. *Intersectoral linkages and health development.* Geneva, World Health Organization, 1984 (WHO Offset Publication, No. 83).

4. **HALSTEAD, S.B.** et al., ed. *Good health at low cost.* New York, Rockefeller Foundation, 1985.

5. **JOLLY, R. & CORNIA, G.A.** *The impact of world recession on children.* Oxford, Pergamon Press, 1985.

6. **KOHLER, L. & MARTIN, J.,** ed. *Inequalities in health and health care.* Göteborg, The Nordic School of Public Health, 1985.

7. **INTERNATIONAL MONETARY FUND.** *Government financial statistics yearbook 1985.* Washington, DC, 1985.

8. **UNCTAD.** *Trade and development report – 1986.* Geneva, UNCTAD, 1986.

9. **UNDP.** *Adjustment and growth with human development.* Salzburg statement, North-South Round Table. New York, 1986.

10. **UNITED NATIONS ECONOMIC AND SOCIAL COUNCIL.** *Overall socio-economic perspective of the world economy for the year 2000.* Report of the Secretary-General. Document 1985/102, 4 June 1985.

11. **UNICEF.** *Within human reach. A future for Africa's children.* New York, 1985.

12. **UNICEF.** *The state of the world's children – 1984, 1985, 1986, 1987.* New York, Oxford University Press, 1984-1987.

13. **UNITED NATIONS.** *National accounts statistics, main aggregates and detailed tables, 1982, and computer tapes.* New York, United Nations, 1985.

14. **WORLD BANK.** *World development report 1985* and *1986.* New York, Oxford University Press, 1985 and 1986.

15. **WHO.** *The role of health economics in national health planning and policy making.* Copenhagen, WHO Regional Office for Europe, 1987.

16. **WHO.** *Global Strategy for Health for All.* Geneva, World Health Organization, 1981 *("Health for All" Series,* No. 3).

17. **ABEL-SMITH, B.** Cost-containment in 12 European countries. *World health statistics quarterly,* **37**: 351-363 (1984).

18. **WHO.** *Repercussions of the world economic recession* – Provisional report by the Director-General. Geneva, WHO, 1986 (document A39/4).

19. **WHO.** *Evaluation of the strategy for health for all by the year 2000. Seventh report on the world health situation. Volume I: Global review.* Geneva, WHO, 1987.

Chapter II

1. *Plan financiero maestro para el plan quinquenal 1986-1990.* Caja Costariccense de Seguro Social, San José, Costa Rica, 1986.

2. **CUMPER, G.** The costs of primary health care. *Tropical doctor,* **14**: 19-22 (1984).

3. **DRUMMOND, M.F. & STODDART, G.L.** Principles of economic evaluation of health programmes. *World health statistics quarterly,* **38** (4): (1985).

4. **GRIFITHS, A. & MILLS, M.** *Money for health: A manual for survey in developing countries.* Geneva, Sandoz Institute for Health and Socio-economic Studies and Ministry of Health, Botswana, 1982.

5. **LAGERGREN, M.** Sweden's plan for 2000. *World health,* May 1986, pp. 7-9.

6. **LEE, K. & MILLS, A.,** ed. *The economics of health in developing countries.* Oxford, Oxford University Press, 1983.

7. **MACH, E.P. & ABEL-SMITH, B.** *Planning the finances of the health sector: A manual for developing countries.* Geneva, WHO, 1985.

8. **MERKLE, A.** *The cost of health for all. A feasibility study from Upper Volta.* Eschborn, German Agency for Technical Development, 1982.

9. **MWABU, G.** *Financial health planning, Kenya (Nairobi, 1986).* Draft paper for the Technical Discussions at the Fortieth World Health Assembly, 1987.

10. *Financial survey of health and social welfare 1987, including a cost estimate 1987-1990,* Health for all by 2000 policy document. The Hague, Ministry of Welfare, Health and Cultural Affairs, 1986.

11. **PARET, H.** *Planification de la santé en Afrique.* Paris, L'Harmettan, 1984.

12. **PUBLIC FINANCE INTERNATIONAL.** *Financial management in the health sector of developing countries.* Background paper for the World Bank. London, Public Finance International, 1982.

13. **THOMAS, M.** *Problems of recurrent costs in the health of developing countries.* Unpublished WHO/SHS document, 1987.

14. **WHO.** *Managerial process for national health development. Guiding principles.* Geneva, World Health Organization, 1981 ("Health for All" Series, No. 5).

15. **WHO.** *Guidelines for costing primary health care development.* Unpublished WHO document, SHS/84.3, 1984.

16. **KLECZKOWSKI, B. et al.** *National health systems and their reorientation towards health for all. Guidance for policy-making.* Geneva, World Health Organization, 1984 (Public Health Papers, No. 77).

17. **KLECZKOWSKI, B. et al.** *Health system support for primary health care.* Geneva, World Health Organization, 1984 (Public Health Papers, No. 80).

18. **WHO.** *Financial planning for Health for All by the Year 2000.* New Delhi, WHO Regional Office for South-East Asia, 1984.

19. **WHO.** *Programme budgeting as part of the managerial process for national health development. Guiding principles.* Unpublished WHO document, MPNHD/84.2, 1984.

20. **WHO.** *Planning of the finances of Health for All.* Report by the Director-General. Geneva, WHO, 1985 (document EB77/INF.DOC./1).

21. **UNICEF/WHO.** *National decision-making for primary health care.* Geneva, WHO, 1981.

22. **WILSON, R.F. et al.** *Planning and management of primary health care programmes. Report of a Workshop.* Geneva, The Aga Khan Foundation, 1984.

Chapter III

1. **COMMONWEALTH.** *Development cooperation for health in Commonwealth countries. Part I and II – Meeting reports, Nassau, The Bahamas, 13-17 October 1986.*

2. **CUMPER, G.** *Health sector financing, estimating health financing in developing countries.* London, London School of Hygiene and Tropical Medicine, 1986.

3. **de FERRANTI, D.** Strategies for paying for health services in developing countries. *World health statistics quarterly,* **37**: 428-450 (1984).

4. **GROSS, P.N. et al.** Revolving drug funds: concluding business in the public sector. *Social science and medicine,* **22**: 335-343 (1986).

5. **KAL HONG PHUA.** Singapore's family saving scheme. *World health,* May 1986, pp. 11-12.

6. **MUSGROVE, P.** What should consumers in poor countries pay for publicly-provided health services? *Social science and medicine,* **22**: 329-333 (1986).

7. **MWABU, G.M. & MWANGI, W.M.** Health care financing in Kenya – A simulation of welfare effects of user fees. *Social science and medicine,* **22**: 763-767 (1986).

8. **OK RYUN MOON.** Towards equity in health care. *World health,* May 1986, p. 20.

9. **RUSSELL, S.S. & REYNOLDS, R.J.** *Community financing.* PRICOR, USA, 1985 (PRICOR Monograph Series, Issues Paper 1).

10. **RUSSELL, S.S. & ZSCHOCK, D.K.** *Health care financing in Latin America and the Caribbean.* New York, HOFLAC, State University of New York, 1986 (Research Report No. 1).

11. **SENE, P.M.** Community financing in Senegal, *World health,* May 1986, pp. 4-5.

12. **SHEPARD, D.S. & BENJAMIN, E.R.** *Mobilizing resources for health. User fees and health financing in developing countries.* Paper for the second Takemi Symposium on International Health. Boston, Harvard School of Public Health, 1986.

13. **STINSON, W.** *Community financing of primary health care.* Washington, DC, American Public Health Associates, 1982 (Primary Health Care Issues, Series 1, No. 4).

14. **WHO.** *Guidelines for preparation of the country health resource. Utilization review document.* Unpublished WHO document, COR/HRG/82.1, 1982.

Chapter IV

1. **ABEL-SMITH, B.** Cost-containment in 12 European countries. *World health statistics quarterly,* **37**: 351-363 (1984).

2. **AMERICAN PUBLIC HEALTH ASSOCIATION.** *Primary health care: progress and problems.* An analysis of 52 projects, assisted by the Agency for International Development of the United States. Washington, DC, 1982.

3. **BANKOWSKI, Z. & FULOP, T.** *Health manpower out of balance: conflicts and prospects.* Geneva, Council for International Organization of Medical Sciences, 1987.

4. **BARNUM, H.N.** Cost-savings from alternative treatment of tuberculosis. Washington, DC, World Bank, 1986 (PHC Technical Note No. 86.11).

5. **BLANPAIN, J.E.** Cost-containment has already been achieved in some countries. *World health forum,* **6**: 11 (1985).

6. **BLUMENFELD, S.N.** *Operations research methods: A general approach in primary health care.* PRICOR, USA, 1985 (PRICOR Monograph Series. Methods Paper 1).

7. **CATSAMBUS, T. & FOSTER, S.** Spending money sensibly: the case of essential drugs. *Finance and development,* **23**: 30-32 (1986).

8. **CREESE, A.L. & HENDERSON, R.H.** Cost-benefit analyses and immunization programmes in developing countries. *Bulletin of the World Health Organization,* **58**: pp. 491-497 (1984).

9. **CULYER, A.J. & HORISBERGER, B.** *Economic and medical evaluation of health care technologies.* Heidelberg, Springer Verlag, 1983.

10. **DRUMMOND, M.F. & MILLS, A.** *Survey of cost-effectiveness and cost-benefit analyses of key primary health care projects in Commonwealth countries.* Commonwealth Secretariat, London, 1986.

11. **EDSTROM, K.** Assessment of the expansion phase in Beheira Government/UNICEF-supported Dayas training programme in Egypt, 1986.

12. **GOLOVOTEEV, V.V. & PUSTOVOJ, I.V.** Public health finance and planning in the Soviet Union. *World health statistics quarterly,* **37**: 364-374 (1984).

13. **GROSSE, R.N. & PLESSES, D.J.** Counting the cost of primary health care. *World health forum,* **5**: 226-230 (1984).

14. **GWATKIN, D.R. et al.** *Can health and nutrition interventions make a difference?* Overseas Development Council Monograph, No. 13, 1983.

15. **JORDAN, P.** *Schistosomiasis: comparison of control strategies.* Cambridge, Cambridge University Press, 1985.

16. **KAEWSONTHI, S.** *Cost and performance appraisal of malaria surveillance and monitoring measures.* Final Report of the UNDP/World Bank/WHO/TDR Project, No. 800435, 1983.

17. **MILLS, A.** Economic evaluation of health programmes – Application of the principles in developing countries. *World health statistics quarterly,* **38**: (1985).

18. **MILLS, A. & THOMAS, M.** *Economic evaluation of health programmes in developing countries. A review and selected annotated bibliography.* London, London School of Hygiene and Tropical Medicine, 1984.

19. **OVER, M.** The effect of scale on cost projections for a primary health care programme in a developing country. *Social science and medicine.* **22**: 351-360 (1986).

20. **PAUL, S.** *Managing development programme: the lessons of success.* Boulder, CO, Westview Special Studies, 1982.

21. **PIACHAUD, D.** Medical equipment in Third World countries. *Journal of tropical medicine and hygiene,* **85**: 183-185 (1982).

22. **REYNOLDS, J. & GASPARI, K.C.** Cost-effectiveness analysis. PRICOR, USA, 1985 (PRICOR Monograph Series, Methods Paper 2).

23. **ROBERTSON, L. et al.** Service volume and other factors affecting the costs of immunizations in The Gambia. *Bulletin of the World Health Organization,* **62**: 729-736 (1984).

24. **SCHIEBER, G.J.** *The financing and delivery of health care in OECD countries: past, present and future.* OECD Report, Tokyo, 25-28 November 1985.

25. **WALSH, J.A. & WARREN, K.** *Strategies for primary health care. Technologies appropriate for the control of disease in the developing world.* Chicago, University of Chicago Press, 1986.

26. **CREESE, A.** EPI – Programme costing guidelines. *Weekly epidemiological record,* **55**: 281-288 (1980).

27. **WHO.** *Guidelines for health care practice in relation to cost-effectiveness.* Copenhagen, WHO Regional Office for Europe, 1981 (Reports and Studies, No. 53).

28. **WHO.** *Control of health care costs in social security systems.* Copenhagen, WHO Regional Office for Europe, 1982 (Reports and Studies, No. 55).

29. **WHO.** *Drug policies and management: procurement and financing of essential drugs.* Report of a Meeting, Madrid, 22-26 October 1984. Unpublished WHO document, DAP/84.5, 1984.

30. **WHO.** *Kenya: rural drug distribution programme. The new drug management system for rural health facilities, Kenya.* Unpublished WHO document, 1985.

31. **WHO.** *Financial and economic aspects of environmental management and its kost-effectiveness as vector control measures.* Draft report of the Sixth Annual Meeting of the panel of

experts on environmental management in vector control, 7-12 September 1986, Geneva.

32. **WORLD BANK.** *World development report – 1985.* Washington, DC, World Bank, 1985.

Chapter V

1. **ALFILER, M.C.** *Partnership and responsibility in financing health activities in the Philippines.* Draft report for the Technical Discussions at the Fortieth World Health Assembly, 1987.

2. **BERCHE, T.** A propos d'une O.N.G. de développement sanitaire: L'Eglise catholique en Afrique et les soins de santé primaires. *Sciences sociales et santé,* **III** (3-4): (1985).

3. **DAVIS, K.** *Recurrent health cost issues related to effectiveness and equity: the US experience.* Draft paper for the Technical Discussions at the Fortieth World Health Assembly, 1987.

4. **MAHLER, H.** The meaning of "Health for All by the Year 2000". *World health forum,* **2**: 8 (1981).

5. **MWABU, G.M.** Health care decisions at the household level: results of a rural health survey. *Social science and medicine,* **23** (3): (1986).

6. **ROEMER, M.** Private medical practice: obstacle to health for all. *World health forum,* **5**: 195-211 (1984).

7. **RONDINELLI, D.A. et al.** *Decentralization in developing countries.* Washington, DC, World Bank (Staff Working Paper, No. 581, Management and Development Series, No. 8).

8. *Promoting health, preventing disease, objectives for the nation.* Department of Health and Human Services, Washington, DC, 1980 (reprinted 1984).

9. **von THUN, F. & ULLRICH, G.J.,** ed. *Fighting rural poverty through self-help: International Conference Report.* Feldafing, Deutsche Stiftung für Internationale Entwicklung, 1985.

10. *Planning for equity in health. A sector review and policy statement.* Harare, Ministry of Health, 1986.

11. **WHO.** *Collaboration with nongovernmental organizations in implementing the Global Strategy for Health for All.* Background document for the Technical discussions at the Thirty-eighth World Health Assembly, 1985 (A38/Technical Discussions/1).

Officers of the technical discussions

General Chairman and Keynote Speaker:

Dr A. Neri, President, Comisión Nacional para el Proyecto Patagonia y Capital, Buenos Aires, Argentina.

Opening Plenary Panel Members:

Dr S. Surjaningrat, Minister of Health, Jakarta, Indonesia
Mr T. Bencheikh, Minister of Public Health, Rabat, Morocco
Dr A.D. Chiduo, Minister for Health and Social Welfare, Dar es Salaam,
    United Republic of Tanzania
Professor B. Abel-Smith, London School of Economics and Political Science,
    London, England

Secretary:	Dr S. Khanna, Director, Health for All Strategy Coordination, WHO, Geneva, Switzerland
Co-Secretary:	Dr M. Jancloes, Medical Officer, Health for All Strategy Coordination, WHO, Geneva, Switzerland

There were four working groups:

Group 1   Economic policies for equity in health

Moderator:	Dr J.O. Norbom, General Secretary, Ministry of Health and Social Affairs, Oslo, Norway
Co-Moderator:	Dr H. Singh, Health Adviser, Planning Commission, New Delhi, India
Experts:	Dr Amorn Nondasuta, Senior Adviser, Ministry of Public Health, Bangkok, Thailand Mr T. Bencheikh, Minister of Public Health, Rabat, Morocco
Secretary:	Dr A. El Bindari Hammad, Intersectoral Cooperation, Division of Strengthening of Health Services, WHO, Geneva, Switzerland
Co-Secretaries:	Mr C. Krishnamurthi, WHO Regional Office for South-East Asia, New Delhi, India Dr C. Vieira, WHO Regional Office for the Americas, Washington, DC, USA Dr H. Hellberg, Director, Division of Public Information and Education for Health, WHO, Geneva, Switzerland

Group 2   Financial planning

Moderator: Mr Mohamed El-Emadi, Minister of Economy and Trade, Damascus, Syrian Arab Republic

Co-Moderator: Professor B. Abel-Smith, London School of Economics and Political Science, London, England

Experts: Professor D. Jolly, Director of Hospital Planning, Assistance publique des Hôpitaux de Paris, Paris, France
Professor Manupendra Malla, Member of the National Planning Commission, Kathmandu, Nepal

Secretary: Mr A. Creese, National Health Systems and Policies, Division of Strengthening of Health Services, WHO, Geneva, Switzerland

Co-Secretaries: Dr C. Vukmanovic, Managerial Process for National Health Development, WHO, Geneva, Switzerland
Mrs S. Ray-Tabona, Office of the Director-General, WHO, Geneva, Switzerland

Group 3   Resources mobilization

Moderator: Professor O. Ransome Kuti, Minister of Health, Lagos, Nigeria

Co-Moderator: Dr G. Miranda Gutierrez, Director, Social Security, Ministry of Health, San José, Costa Rica

Experts: Professor M. Concepcion Alfiler, Associate Professor, College of Public Administration, University of the Philippines, Philippines
Mr S. Kananiye, Economist, Member of the National Assembly, Bujumbura, Burundi

Secretary: Dr S. Kingma, Health Resources Mobilization, Programme for External Coordination, WHO, Geneva, Switzerland

Co-Secretaries: Dr H. Zöllner, WHO Regional Office for Europe, Copenhagen, Denmark
Mr L. Laugeri, Community Water Supply and Sanitation, Division of Environmental Health, WHO, Geneva, Switzerland
Mr F. Golladay, World Bank, Washington, USA

Group 4   Making better use of resources

Moderator: Dr M. Kökény, Health Policy Adviser to the Deputy Prime Minister, Budapest, Hungary

Co-Moderator:	Dr A. Khalid bin Sahan, Director-General of Health, Ministry of Health, Kuala Lumpur, Malaysia
Experts:	Professor R. Andreano, Department of Economics, University of Wisconsin, USA
	Dr G. Mwabu, Institute of Development Studies, University of Nairobi, Kenya
Secretary:	Dr S. Sapirie, Division of Family Health, WHO, Geneva, Switzerland
Co-Secretaries:	Dr Omer Imam Omer, WHO Regional Office for the Eastern Mediterranean, Alexandria, Egypt
	Dr J. Martin, District Health Systems, Division of Strengthening of Health Services, WHO, Geneva, Switzerland
	Dr N. Drager, Health Resources Mobilization, Programme for External Coordination, WHO, Geneva, Switzerland

Acknowledgements

The preparatory work for this publication included studies, consultations, and meetings; funds to support these were provided by the Belgian Government, the Gruppo Volontariato Civile, Bologna, Italy, the French Government, the Pew Foundation, the Rockefeller Foundation, the Fondation Rhône-Poulenc Santé, and the United States Agency for International Development.

The technical assistance of Mr F. Golladay, economist at the World Bank, is gratefully acknowledged.

Thanks are also due to the following people who provided material for the discussions and background documents: Professor B. Abel-Smith, London School of Economics and Political Science, London, England; Mrs S. Abramson, USAID, Washington, DC, USA; Mr J. Akin, World Bank, Washington, DC, USA; Professor Brunet-Jailly, Ecole de Recherche en Santé publique, Bamako, Mali; Mr G.A. Cornia, UNICEF, New York, USA; Mr D. Gwatkin, Pew Foundation, Washington, USA; Dr A. Khalid bin Sahan, Director General of Health, Ministry of Health, Kuala Lumpur, Malaysia; Mr B. Lanvin, Office of the Secretary-General, UNCTAD, Geneva, Switzerland; Dr G. Miranda Gutierrez, Director, Social Security, Ministry of Health, San José, Costa Rica; Dr A. Neri, Comisión Nacional para el Proyecto Patagonia y Capital, Buenos Aires, Argentina; Dr G. Mwabu, University of Nairobi, Nairobi, Kenya; Mr Tamburi, Department of Social Security, ILO, Geneva, Switzerland, Mrs A. Tinker, Health Services Division, USAID, Washington, USA; Dr K. Warren, Division of Health Sciences, Rockefeller Foundation, New York, USA.

The following WHO staff members assisted the Secretariat in preparing for the discussions: Mr A. Creese, National Health Systems and Policies, Division of Strengthening of Health Services; Dr A. El Bindari Hammad, Intersectoral Cooperation, Division of Strengthening of Health Services; Dr H. Hellberg, Division of Public Information and Education for Health; Dr S. Kingma, Health Resources Mobilization, Programme for External Coordination; Mr L. Laugeri, Community Water Supply and Sanitation, Division of Environmental Health; Dr Maitu, District Health Systems, Division of Strengthening of Health Services; Mrs S. Ray-Tabona, Office of the Director-General; Dr P. Rosenfield, Social and Economic Research, Special Programme for Research and Training in Tropical Diseases; Dr S. Sapirie, Division of Family Health; Mrs M. Thomas, Division of Noncommunicable Diseases; Dr C. Vukmanovic, Managerial Process for National Health Development; Dr O.I. Omer, Health Manpower Development, WHO Regional Office for the Eastern Mediterranean, Alexandria, Egypt; and Dr H. Zollner, Health Economics, WHO Regional Office for Europe, Copenhagen, Denmark.

WHO publications may be obtained, direct or through booksellers, from:

ALGERIA: Entreprise nationale du Livre (ENAL), 3 bd Zirout Youcef, ALGIERS

ARGENTINA: Carlos Hirsch, SRL, Florida 165, Galerías Güemes, Escritorio 453/465, BUENOS AIRES

AUSTRALIA: Hunter Publications, 58A Gipps Street, COLLINGWOOD, VIC 3066.

AUSTRIA: Gerold & Co., Graben 31, 1011 VIENNA I

BAHRAIN: United Schools International, Arab Region Office, P.O. Box 726, BAHRAIN

BANGLADESH: The WHO Representative, G.P.O. Box 250, DHAKA 5

BELGIUM: *For books:* Office International de Librairie s.a., avenue Marnix 30, 1050 BRUSSELS. *For periodicals and subscriptions:* Office International des Périodiques, avenue Louise 485, 1050 BRUSSELS.

BHUTAN: *see* India, WHO Regional Office

BOTSWANA: Botsalo Books (Pty) Ltd., P.O. Box 1532, GABORONE

BRAZIL: Centro Latinoamericano de Informação em Ciencias de Saúde (BIREME), Organização Panamericana de Saúde, Sector de Publicações, C.P. 20381 - Rua Botucatu 862, 04023 SÃO PAULO, SP

BURMA: *see* India, WHO Regional Office

CAMEROON: Cameroon Book Centre, P.O. Box 123, South West Province, VICTORIA

CANADA: Canadian Public Health Association, 1335 Carling Avenue, Suite 210, OTTAWA, Ont. K1Z 8N8. (Tel: (613) 725–3769. Telex: 21–053–3841)

CHINA: China National Publications Import & Export Corporation, P.O. Box 88, BEIJING (PEKING)

DEMOCRATIC PEOPLE'S REPUBLIC OF KOREA: *see* India, WHO Regional Office

DENMARK: Munksgaard Export and Subscription Service, Nørre Søgade 35, 1370 COPENHAGEN K (Tel: + 45 1 12 85 70)

FIJI: The WHO Representative, P.O. Box 113, SUVA

FINLAND: Akateeminen Kirjakauppa, Keskuskatu 2, 00101 HELSINKI 10

FRANCE: Arnette, 2 rue Casimir-Delavigne, 75006 PARIS

GERMAN DEMOCRATIC REPUBLIC: Buchhaus Leipzig, Postfach 140, 701 LEIPZIG

GERMANY FEDERAL REPUBLIC OF: Govi-Verlag GmbH, Ginnheimerstrasse 20, Postfach 5360, 6236 ESCHBORN — Buchhandlung Alexander Horn, Kirchgasse 22, Postfach 3340, 6200 WIESBADEN

GREECE: G.C. Eleftheroudakis S.A., Librairie internationale, rue Nikis 4, 105-63 ATHENS

HONG KONG: Hong Kong Government Information Services, Publication (Sales) Office, Information Services Department, No. 1, Battery Path, Central, HONG KONG.

HUNGARY: Kultura, P.O.B. 149, BUDAPEST 62

ICELAND: Snaebjorn Jonsson & Co., Hafnarstraeti 9, P.O. Box 1131, IS-101 REYKJAVIK

INDIA: WHO Regional Office for South-East Asia, World Health House, Indraprastha Estate, Mahatma Gandhi Road, NEW DELHI 110002

IRAN (ISLAMIC REPUBLIC OF): Iran University Press, 85 Park Avenue, P.O. Box 54/551, TEHRAN

IRELAND: TDC Publishers, 12 North Frederick Street, DUBLIN 1 (Tel: 744835–749677)

ISRAEL: Heiliger & Co., 3 Nathan Strauss Street, JERUSALEM 94227

ITALY: Edizioni Minerva Medica, Corso Bramante 83–85, 10126 TURIN; Via Lamarmora 3, 20100 MILAN; Via Spallanzani 9, 00161 ROME

JAPAN: Maruzen Co. Ltd., P.O. Box 5050, TOKYO International, 100–31

JORDAN: Jordan Book Centre Co. Ltd., University Street, P.O. Box 301 (Al-Jubeiha), AMMAN

KENYA: Text Book Centre Ltd, P.O. Box 47540, NAIROBI

KUWAIT: The Kuwait Bookshops Co. Ltd., Thunayan Al-Ghanem Bldg, P.O. Box 2942, KUWAIT

LAO PEOPLE'S DEMOCRATIC REPUBLIC: The WHO Representative, P.O. Box 343, VIENTIANE

LUXEMBOURG: Librairie du Centre, 49 bd Royal, LUXEMBOURG